WHO recommendations for
augmentation of labour

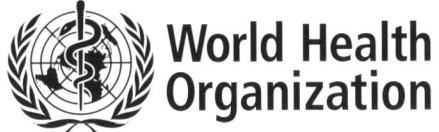

WHO Library Cataloguing-in-Publication Data

WHO recommendations for augmentation of labour.

1.Dystocia – prevention and control. 2.Labor, Induced – methods. 3.Labor, Induced - standards. 4.Labor Presentation. 5.Perinatal Care – methods. 6.Guideline. I.World Health Organization.

ISBN 978 92 4 150736 3 (NLM classification: WQ 440)

© World Health Organization 2014

All rights reserved. Publications of the World Health Organization are available on the WHO website (www.who.int) or can be purchased from WHO Press, World Health Organization, 20 Avenue Appia, 1211 Geneva 27, Switzerland
(tel.: +41 22 791 3264; fax: +41 22 791 4857; e-mail: bookorders@who.int).

Requests for permission to reproduce or translate WHO publications –whether for sale or for non-commercial distribution– should be addressed to WHO Press through the WHO website (www.who.int/about/licensing/copyright_form/en/index.html).

The designations employed and the presentation of the material in this publication do not imply the expression of any opinion whatsoever on the part of the World Health Organization concerning the legal status of any country, territory, city or area or of its authorities, or concerning the delimitation of its frontiers or boundaries. Dotted lines on maps represent approximate border lines for which there may not yet be full agreement.

The mention of specific companies or of certain manufacturers' products does not imply that they are endorsed or recommended by the World Health Organization in preference to others of a similar nature that are not mentioned. Errors and omissions excepted, the names of proprietary products are distinguished by initial capital letters.

All reasonable precautions have been taken by the World Health Organization to verify the information contained in this publication. However, the published material is being distributed without warranty of any kind, either expressed or implied. The responsibility for the interpretation and use of the material lies with the reader. In no event shall the World Health Organization be liable for damages arising from its use.

Printed in France

Table of Contents

Acknowledgements	1
Acronyms and abbreviations	2
Executive summary	3
Introduction	3
Guideline development methods	3
Guiding principles	4
Summary list of WHO recommendations for augmentation of labour	5
1. Background	6
1.1 Target audience	6
2. Methods	7
2.1 Declaration of interests by participants at the WHO technical consultation	8
2.2 Decision-making during the technical consultation	8
2.3 Document preparation and peer review	9
3. Results	9
3.1 Guiding principles	9
3.2 Definition of delay in the first stage of labour	10
3.3 Evidence and recommendations	10
4. Research implications	44
4.1 Key research priorities	44
4.2 Other research questions	44
5. Dissemination and implementation of the guideline	44
5.1 Guideline dissemination and evaluation	44
5.2 Guideline implementation	45
6. Applicability issues	45
6.1 Anticipated impact on the organization of care and resources	45
6.2 Monitoring and evaluating the guideline implementation	45
7. Updating the guideline	46
References	47
Annex 1. External experts and WHO staff involved in the preparation of the guideline	49
Annex 2. Critical and important outcomes for decision-making	52
Annex 3. Summary of the considerations related to the strength of the recommendations (balance worksheets)	53

The standardized criteria used in grading the evidence and GRADE tables are not included in this document although table numbers – prefixed with "EB" for evidence base – are included for ease of reference. The full evidence tables have been published in a separate document entitled *WHO recommendations for augmentation of labour: evidence base,* which can be accessed online at www.who.int/reproductivehealth/topics/maternal_perinatal/augmentation-labour.

Acknowledgements

Work on this guideline was initiated by A. Metin Gülmezoglu, João Paulo Souza and Mariana Widmer, of the WHO Department of Reproductive Health and Research, and Matthews Mathai, of the WHO Department of Maternal, Newborn, Child and Adolescent Health. Olufemi Oladapo, of the WHO Department of Reproductive Health and Research, coordinated the development of the guideline and drafted this document. Therese Dowswell and Helen West, of the Cochrane Pregnancy and Childbirth Group, University of Liverpool, United Kingdom, reviewed the scientific evidence related to augmentation of labour, prepared the GRADE tables and drafted the narrative summaries of evidence used in this guideline. Sonja Henderson, also of the Cochrane Pregnancy and Childbirth Group, University of Liverpool, United Kingdom, coordinated the updating of relevant Cochrane reviews and review of the scientific evidence. The GRADE tables were double-checked by Olufemi Oladapo. A. Metin Gülmezoglu, João Paulo Souza and Matthews Mathai commented on the draft document before it was reviewed by participants at the WHO technical consultation on augmentation of labour and external reviewers.

WHO extends sincere thanks to Zahida Qureshi, of the University of Nairobi, Kenya, for chairing the technical consultation. We acknowledge the valuable feedback provided by a large number of international stakeholders during the online consultation, which took place before the meeting, as part of the guideline development process.

WHO gratefully acknowledges the continued support of the United States Agency for International Development (USAID) in this area of work. Special thanks are due to the authors of the systematic reviews used in this guideline for their assistance and collaboration in updating the reviews. WHO is also grateful to the Cochrane Pregnancy and Childbirth Group, especially the staff at their Liverpool office in the United Kingdom, for their support in updating the Cochrane reviews.

Acronyms and abbreviations

CI	confidence interval
EB	evidence base
FWC	Family, Women's and Children's Health (a WHO cluster)
GDG	Guideline Development Group
GRADE	Grading of Recommendations Assessment, Development and Evaluation
GREAT	Guideline development, Research priorities, Evidence synthesis, Applicability of evidence, Transfer of knowledge (a WHO project)
hr	hour
IM	intramuscular
IV	intravenous
MCA	[WHO Department of] Maternal, Newborn, Child and Adolescent Health
mcg	microgram
MD	mean difference
min	minute
ml	millilitre
MPA	Maternal and Perinatal Health & Preventing Unsafe Abortion (a team in WHO's Department of Reproductive Health and Research)
NICU	neonatal intensive care unit
PPH	postpartum haemorrhage
RCT	randomized controlled trial
RHR	[WHO Department of] Reproductive Health and Research
RR	relative risk
TENS	transcutaneous electrical nerve stimulation
WHO	World Health Organization

Executive summary

Introduction

Prolonged labour is an important cause of maternal and perinatal mortality and morbidity. Common underlying causes include inefficient uterine contractions, abnormal fetal presentation or position, inadequate bony pelvis or soft tissue abnormalities of the mother. Identifying the exact cause of slowly progressing labour in clinical practice can be challenging. Thus, "failure of labour to progress" has become one of the leading indications for primary caesarean section, particularly in first-time mothers. There is growing concern that caesarean section is performed too soon in many cases, without exploring less invasive interventions that could lead to vaginal birth.

Augmentation of labour is the process of stimulating the uterus to increase the frequency, duration and intensity of contractions after the onset of spontaneous labour. It has commonly been used to treat delayed labour when poor uterine contractions are assessed to be the underlying cause. The traditional methods of labour augmentation have been with the use of intravenous oxytocin infusion and artificial rupture of the membranes (amniotomy). Over the last few decades, efforts to avoid prolonged labour in institutional birth have led to the use of a range of practices to either accelerate slow labour or drive the physiological process of normally progressing labour. While interventions within the context of augmentation of labour may be beneficial, their inappropriate use can cause harm. Besides, unnecessary clinical intervention in the natural birth process undermines women's autonomy and dignity as recipients of care and may negatively impact their childbirth experience.

Optimizing outcomes for women in labour at the global level requires evidence-based guidance of health workers to improve care through appropriate patient selection and use of effective interventions. In this regard, the World Health Organization (WHO) published recommendations for induction of labour in 2011. The goal of the present guideline is to consolidate the guidance for effective interventions that are needed to reduce the global burden of prolonged labour and its consequences. The primary target audience includes health professionals responsible for developing national and local health protocols and policies, as well as obstetricians, midwives, nurses, general medical practitioners, managers of maternal and child health programmes, and public health policy-makers in all settings.

Guideline development methods

This guideline was developed in accordance with the procedures outlined in the *WHO handbook for guideline development*. These involved: (i) identification of priority questions and critical outcomes, (ii) retrieval of up-to-date evidence, (iii) assessment and synthesis of the evidence, (iv) formulation of recommendations using input from a wide range of stakeholders, and (v) planning for the dissemination, implementation, impact evaluation and updating of the guideline.

The scientific evidence for the recommendations was synthesized using the Grading of Recommendations Assessment, Development and Evaluation (GRADE) methodology. For the prioritized questions, evidence profiles were prepared based on up-to-date systematic reviews. Based on the evidence profiles, the recommendations were formulated and approved by an international group of experts who participated in the WHO technical consultation on augmentation of labour, held in Geneva, Switzerland, on 26–27 September 2013.

The WHO technical consultation adopted 20 recommendations covering practices relating to the diagnosis, prevention and treatment of delayed progress in the first stage of labour, and supportive care for women undergoing labour augmentation. For each recommendation, the quality of the supporting evidence was graded as very low, low, moderate or high. The contributing experts qualified the strength of these recommendations (as strong or weak) by considering the quality of the evidence and other factors, including values and preferences of stakeholders, the magnitude of effect, the balance of benefits versus harms, resource use and the feasibility of each recommendation. To ensure that each recommendation is correctly understood and used in practice, additional remarks and an evidence summary have also been prepared, and these are provided in the full document, below each recommendation. Guideline users should refer to this information in the full version of the guideline if they are in any doubt as to the basis for any of the recommendations.

Guiding principles

The participants at the technical consultation agreed that the following overarching principles are applicable to all the recommendations in this guideline. These principles were consensus-based and were not derived from a systematic process of evidence retrieval, synthesis and grading. They are intended to underscore the importance of respect for women's rights and dignity as recipients of care, and the need to maintain high ethical and safety standards in clinical practice. The principles are not by themselves specific recommendations but are expected to guide end-users in the process of adapting and implementing the guideline in a range of contexts and settings.

- Application of the recommendations should be based on consideration of the general condition of the woman and her baby, her wishes and preferences, and respect for her dignity and autonomy.

- Augmentation of labour should be performed only when there is a clear medical indication and the expected benefits outweigh the potential harms.

- Women undergoing augmentation of labour, particularly with oxytocin, should not be left unattended.

- Augmentation of labour with oxytocin is appropriate and should only be performed after conducting clinical assessment to exclude cephalopelvic disproportion. This principle is relevant for all women but is even more crucial for multiparous women.

- As the evidence for these recommendations was largely informed by studies conducted among women with pregnancies in cephalic presentation and unscarred uterus, they should not be applied to women with abnormal fetal presentation (including breech) or scarred uterus.

- Augmentation of labour should be performed with caution as the procedure carries the risk of uterine hyperstimulation, with the potential consequences of fetal distress and uterine rupture.

- Wherever augmentation of labour is performed, facilities should be available to closely and regularly monitor fetal heart rate and uterine contraction pattern.

- Augmentation of labour should be carried out in facilities where there is capacity to manage its potential outcomes, including adverse effects and failure to achieve vaginal birth.

Summary list of WHO recommendations for augmentation of labour

This table contains specific recommendations as formulated and approved by participants at the WHO technical consultation on augmentation of labour.

Context	Recommendation	Quality of evidence	Strength of recommendation
Diagnosis of delay in the first stage of labour	1. Active phase partograph with a four-hour action line is recommended for monitoring the progress of labour.	Very low	Strong
	2. Digital vaginal examination at intervals of four hours is recommended for routine assessment and identification of delay in active labour.	Very low	Weak
Prevention of delay in the first stage of labour	3. A package of care for active management of labour for prevention of delay in labour is not recommended.	Low	Weak
	4. The use of early amniotomy with early oxytocin augmentation for prevention of delay in labour is not recommended.	Very low	Weak
	5. The use of oxytocin for prevention of delay in labour in women receiving epidural analgesia is not recommended.	Low	Weak
	6. The use of amniotomy alone for prevention of delay in labour is not recommended.	Very low	Weak
	7. The use of antispasmodic agents for prevention of delay in labour is not recommended.	Very low	Weak
	8. Pain relief for preventing delay and reducing the use of augmentation in labour is not recommended.	Very low	Weak
	9. The use of intravenous fluids with the aim of shortening the duration of labour is not recommended.	Very low	Strong
	10. For women at low risk, oral fluid and food intake during labour is recommended.	Very low	Weak
	11. Encouraging the adoption of mobility and upright position during labour in women at low risk is recommended.	Very low	Strong
	12. Continuous companionship during labour is recommended for improving labour outcomes.	Moderate	Strong
	13. Administration of enema for reducing the use of labour augmentation is not recommended.	Very low	Strong
Treatment of delay in the first stage of labour with augmentation	14. The use of oxytocin alone for treatment of delay in labour is recommended.	Very low	Weak
	15. Augmentation with intravenous oxytocin prior to confirmation of delay in labour is not recommended.	Very low	Weak
	16. High starting and increment dosage regimen of oxytocin is not recommended for labour augmentation.	Very low	Weak
	17. The use of oral misoprostol for labour augmentation is not recommended.	Very low	Strong
	18. The use of amniotomy alone for treatment of delay in labour is not recommended.	Very low	Weak
	19. The use of amniotomy and oxytocin for treatment of confirmed delay in labour is recommended.	Very low	Weak
Care during labour augmentation	20. The use of internal tocodynamometry, compared with external tocodynamometry, with the aim of improving outcomes for augmented labour is not recommended.	Very low	Weak

1. Background

Difficult labour (or dystocia) is characterized by abnormally slow labour progress arising from inefficient uterine contractions, abnormal fetal presentation or position, inadequate bony pelvis or abnormalities of the pelvic soft tissues of the mother. It is more common among nulliparous women and is associated with considerable maternal and perinatal morbidity and mortality as a result of infections, uterine rupture and operative deliveries *(1, 2)*. As a result of lack of universal consensus about what defines delay in the first stage of labour, the incidence is not accurately known. Some evidence suggests that up to one third of first-time mothers experience delay in the first stage of labour *(3)*.

In clinical practice, identifying the precise cause of slow labour progress can be challenging. Thus, "failure to progress" has become an increasingly popular description of delayed labour and one of the leading indications for primary caesarean section *(4)*. There is growing concern that caesarean section is performed too soon in many cases, without due consideration for less invasive interventions that could lead to vaginal birth.

Augmentation of labour is the process of stimulating the uterus to increase the frequency, duration and intensity of contractions after the onset of spontaneous labour. It has commonly been used to treat delayed labour when uterine contractions are assessed to be insufficiently strong or inappropriately coordinated to dilate the cervix. Labour augmentation has traditionally been performed with the use of intravenous oxytocin infusion and/or artificial rupture of amniotic membranes (amniotomy). The procedure aims to shorten labour in order to prevent complications relating to undue prolongation, and to avert caesarean section. It is central to the concept of active management of the first stage of labour, which was proposed more than four decades ago as a strategy for expediting labour and reducing caesarean section rates *(5)*. Active management of labour as originally proposed was based on the philosophy that there were benefits in actively driving the natural labour process, although continuous one-to-one care as one of its components is often not followed through in practice *(6)*.

In spite of the general rule that labour augmentation with oxytocin should only be performed for valid indications, reports have shown poor adherence to this rule in clinical practice. There is evidence that a significant proportion of women with uncomplicated pregnancies are subjected to routine augmentation of labour with oxytocin *(7)*.

There have also been reports of unstructured use of labour augmentation, where women are given oxytocin inadequately or unnecessarily *(8)*. While augmentation of labour may be beneficial in preventing prolonged labour, its inappropriate use may cause harm. Augmentation with synthetic oxytocin may result in uterine hyperstimulation, with adverse effects such as fetal asphyxia and uterine rupture, and thus increase the risk of a cascade of interventions during labour and delivery *(9)*. Besides, such unwarranted clinical intervention deprives women of their autonomy and dignity during labour and may negatively impact their childbirth experience. The use of herbal remedies with uncertain oxytocic properties for labour induction and augmentation is also widely known.

There is wide disparity in the current practice of oxytocin augmentation between countries and between hospitals in the same country *(10)*. This variation is largely related to the differences in the indications, dosage and timing of initiating oxytocin, use of special procedures (e.g. epidural analgesia), and whether or not and at what point other methods, such as amniotomy, should be included. Available expert guidelines for the practice of labour augmentation are also inconsistent across the range of clinical scenarios. As a common intrapartum intervention, improving the practice of labour augmentation through provision of evidence-informed guidelines has significant implications for labour outcomes in both low- and high-income countries.

For low-income countries to remain on track towards the fifth Millennium Development Goal, evidence-based guidance is required for their health workers to comprehensively improve intrapartum care through appropriate patient selection and use of effective interventions. In this regard, the World Health Organization (WHO) published recommendations for induction of labour – another critical intervention in labour management – in 2011 *(11)*. The goal of the present guideline is to consolidate the guidance for effective interventions related to intrapartum care. It was developed on the premise of ensuring the safety and autonomy of mothers during labour while tackling the global problem of high caesarean section rate.

1.1 Target audience

The primary audience for this guideline includes health professionals responsible for developing national and local health protocols and policies, as well as obstetricians, midwives, nurses, general medical practitioners, managers of maternal and child health programmes, and public health policy-makers in all settings. This guidance is evidence-informed and covers topics related to labour augmentation that were selected and prioritized by an international, multidisciplinary group of health care professionals, consumers and other stakeholders. It provides the general principles and specific recommendations for augmentation of labour and is intended to inform the development of protocols and health policies related to labour augmentation. It is not intended to provide a comprehensive practical guide for augmentation of labour.

2. Methods

This document represents WHO's normative support for using evidence-informed policies and practices in all countries. This guideline forms part of a WHO knowledge-to-action project entitled GREAT (Guideline development, Research priorities, Evidence synthesis, Applicability of evidence, Transfer of knowledge) *(12)* and was developed using standardized operating procedures in accordance with the process described in the *WHO handbook for guideline development (13)*. In summary, the process included: (i) identification of priority questions and critical outcomes, (ii) retrieval of the evidence, (iii) assessment and synthesis of the evidence, (iv) formulation of recommendations, and (v) planning for the dissemination, implementation, impact evaluation and updating of the guideline.

First, a Guideline Steering Group was constituted with WHO staff from the Department of Reproductive Health and Research (RHR) and the Department of Maternal, Newborn, Child and Adolescent Health (MCA). This group drafted a list of questions and outcomes related to augmentation of labour. Then WHO consulted a large group of international stakeholders including midwives, obstetricians, neonatologists, researchers, experts in research synthesis, experts in health care programmes, and consumer representatives to review and prioritize the draft questions and outcomes. From this pool of stakeholders, a Guideline Development Group (GDG) and an External Review Group were set up to support the guideline development process. The GDG was made up of external experts whose tasks were to provide advice on the guideline development process, appraise the evidence used to inform the guidelines, advise on the interpretation of this evidence, and formulate the final recommendations. The main role of the External Review Group was to review and comment on the finalized guideline document. The members of the Guideline Steering Group and the External Review Group are listed in Annex 1.

The large group of international stakeholders rated the questions and outcomes, which had been drafted by the Guideline Steering Group, on a scale from one to nine. In this context, a question or outcome was defined as "critical" if it was given an average score of seven or more. Questions and outcomes with a score of between four and six were considered "important but not critical", while those with a score lower than four were not considered to be important for the purposes of the guideline. The lists of critical and important outcomes are provided in Annex 2. The prioritized questions and the outcomes rated as critical were included in the scope of this document for evidence searching, retrieval, grading and formulation of recommendations. In situations where critical outcomes were poorly reported in a systematic review, "important but not critical" outcomes were used to complement the evidence base for the recommendations.

Cochrane systematic reviews of randomized controlled trials (RCTs) were the primary source of evidence for the recommendations.[1] Using the assembled lists of questions and outcomes, the Guideline Steering Group along with an external team of guideline methodologists (who were also members of the GDG) reviewed the scientific evidence, prepared the evidence profiles, and drafted the narrative summaries of evidence used in this guideline. First, they identified Cochrane systematic reviews that were either relevant or potentially relevant and then assessed whether they needed to be updated. A review was considered to be outdated if the last specified date for new trial searches was two years ago or more, or if there were relevant trials still awaiting assessment, as identified by the standard search procedures of the Cochrane Pregnancy and Childbirth Group. Updates were performed using standard search strategies. For reviews found to be outdated, the contact authors of such reviews were requested to update them within a specified time period. In instances in which the contact authors were unable to do so, the updates were undertaken by the external team of methodologists in consultation with the Guideline Steering Group. The search strategies employed to identify the trials and the specific criteria for trial inclusion and exclusion are described in the individual systematic reviews.

The following procedures were used to extract the evidence for this guideline from each of these systematic

---

1   As part of the Cochrane prepublication editorial process, reviews are commented on by three peers (one editor and two referees external to the editorial team) and the Cochrane review group's statistical adviser. *The Cochrane Handbook for Systematic Reviews of Interventions* describes in detail the process of preparing and maintaining Cochrane systematic reviews on the effects of health care interventions; it is available online at http://handbook.cochrane.org/.

reviews: first, the most up-to-date version of the Review Manager (RevMan) file was obtained from the Cochrane Pregnancy and Childbirth Group and customized to reflect the key comparisons and outcomes (excluding those that were not relevant to the guideline). Then the RevMan file was exported to the GRADE profiler software (Grading of Recommendations Assessment, Development and Evaluation) and the GRADE criteria were applied to critically appraise the retrieved scientific evidence. Finally, evidence profiles (in the form of GRADE tables) were prepared for each comparison. This process was managed through an online collaborative process between the WHO Guideline Steering Group and the external team of guideline methodologists.

The evidence presented in the GRADE tables was derived from a large body of data extracted primarily from Cochrane reviews, which in many cases contained multiple comparisons. Each GRADE table relates to one specific question or comparison, but some GRADE tables do not contain data for all critical outcomes. This is because data for those outcomes were not available in the Cochrane reviews. The raw data that formed the basis of the GRADE tables are not included in this document, but can be made available to readers interested in how these GRADE tables were constructed. The Guideline Steering Group used the information presented in the GRADE tables to draft recommendations related to each question. Each recommendation was allocated to a thematic module, which included the narrative summaries of evidence and the relevant GRADE tables. The standardized criteria used in grading the evidence and the thematic modules (including the GRADE tables themselves) are not included in this document. They have been published separately in a document entitled *WHO recommendations for augmentation of labour: evidence base*.[2]

A preliminary online consultation was held to review the draft recommendations. The draft recommendations and supporting evidence were made available to the members of the GDG and they were asked to comment on the document in tracked mode. Members of the GDG and additional experts from WHO regional offices were then invited to attend the WHO technical consultation on augmentation of labour, held at WHO headquarters in Geneva, Switzerland, on 26–27 September 2013 (see Annex 1 for a full list of participants). The draft recommendations, the narrative summaries of evidence, the GRADE tables for the recommendations, and other related documents were provided to participants in advance. Balance worksheets were used during the technical consultation to summarize the values, preferences and judgements made about the strength of recommendations (see Annex 3, Boxes 1–4 for the summary of considerations relating to the strength of all recommendations, and Box 5 for the explanations underlying the use of the balance worksheets).

2.1 Declaration of interests by participants at the WHO technical consultation

According to WHO regulations, all experts serving in an advisory role must declare their relevant interests prior to participation in WHO meetings. All GDG members and other participants were therefore required to complete a Declaration of Interest form before the technical consultation. The Guideline Steering Group reviewed the group's declarations before invitations were finalized. The GDG members were also asked to verbally declare potential conflicts of interest at the beginning of the meeting. The procedures for the management of conflicts of interest were undertaken in accordance with the *WHO guidelines for declaration of interests (WHO experts)*. In summary, all members of the GDG declared that they had no academic, commercial or financial interests that were directly or indirectly related to the subject to be discussed at the meeting. Full participation of all the selected experts was deemed appropriate.

2.2 Decision-making during the technical consultation

The technical consultation process was guided by the following protocol: the meeting was designed to allow participants to discuss each of the recommendations drafted by the Guideline Steering Group. Where necessary, each of these recommendations was revised through group discussion. The final adoption of each recommendation was made by consensus – defined as the agreement by at least three quarters of the participants – provided that those who disagreed did not feel strongly about their position. Strong disagreements would have been noted as such in the final guideline, if such events were recorded. When the participants were unable to reach a consensus, the disputed recommendation, or any other decision, was put to a vote. A recommendation or decision stood if a simple majority (more than half of the participants) voted in support of it, unless the disagreement was related to a safety concern, in which case the WHO Secretariat might decide not to issue a recommendation at all. WHO staff, the external methodologists and the observers at the meeting were not eligible to vote. If the issue to be voted upon involved primary research or systematic reviews conducted

---

2 Available at: www.who.int/reproductivehealth/topics/maternal_perinatal/augmentation-labour

by any of the participants who had declared an academic conflict of interest, the participants in question would be allowed to participate in the discussion, but would not be allowed to vote on that particular issue.

The participants at the technical consultation also determined the strength of each recommendation. By default, the strength of each recommendation was aligned initially with the quality of the evidence, such that, at the start of the discussion, strong recommendations were based on evidence that was considered to be of moderate and high quality, while weak recommendations were based on evidence that had been graded as low and very low quality. In addition to evaluating the scientific evidence and its quality, the following factors were also considered when determining the strength and direction of the final recommendation: values and preferences, the magnitude of effect, the balance of benefits versus harms, resource use and feasibility *(14)*. Values and preferences, resource use, and the feasibility of each recommendation were based on the experience and opinions of the GDG members. Balance worksheets were used to note and synthesize these considerations and to record the reasons for changes made to the default strength of the recommendations (see Annex 3). In general, a high quality, strong recommendation indicates that further research on the particular question is not considered to be a priority.

2.3 Document preparation and peer review

Prior to the technical consultation, the Guideline Steering Group prepared a preliminary version of this document using a guideline reporting template that had been developed as part of WHO's GREAT project *(12)*. The draft guideline was made available to the invited participants one week before the meeting for their comments. During the meeting, the draft recommendations were modified in line with participants' deliberation and comments. Feedback received during the preliminary online consultation was also discussed and incorporated into the document where appropriate. After the meeting, members of the Guideline Steering Group worked to ensure that a revised version of the document accurately reflected the deliberations and decisions of the meeting participants. The revised draft guideline document was sent to the members of External Review Group and their inputs were carefully evaluated by the Guideline Steering Group for inclusion in the revised document. After the technical consultation, the Guideline Steering Group refrained from making substantive changes to the guideline scoping (such as the further expansion of the guideline scoping) or to the recommendations. The revised version was returned electronically to those who had participated in the technical consultation for their final approval.

3. Results

Stakeholders from all WHO regions participated in the preliminary online survey. Feedback from the survey was used to modify the recommendation questions and prioritize the outcomes. Annex 2 shows the "critical" and "important" maternal and infant outcomes as rated by the survey participants. In total, 27 Cochrane systematic reviews summarized in 82 GRADE tables provided the evidence base for the 20 recommendations included in this guideline. The recommendations were finalized by the participants at the WHO technical consultation (see Annex 1).

Section 3.1 presents a number of overarching principles, which, according to the assessment of the Guideline Development Group (GDG), are by themselves not specific recommendations but are nonetheless crucial for clear understanding and appropriate implementation of the guideline by end-users. In Section 3.2, the definition of delay in the first stage of labour, which underpinned the consolidation of the evidence base and the formulation of the recommendations, is presented. Section 3.3 presents each of the 20 recommendations, including a narrative summary of the relevant evidence and information about the quality of the evidence and the strength of the recommendation. Additional remarks were also included to ensure that each recommendation is correctly understood and used in practice. The balance worksheets summarizing the values, preferences and judgements made to determine the strength and direction of the recommendations are presented in Annex 3. The corresponding GRADE tables for each of the recommendations are referred to in this section as evidence base (EB) Tables 1 to 20. These tables are presented separately in the supplemental document, *WHO recommendations for augmentation of labour: evidence base*.[3]

3.1 Guiding principles

The participants at the technical consultation agreed that the following overarching principles are applicable to all the recommendations in this guideline. These principles were consensus-based and were not derived from a systematic process of evidence retrieval and synthesis. They are intended to underscore the importance of respect for women's rights and dignity as recipients of care, and the need to maintain high ethical and safety standards in clinical practice. They also draw attention to cross-

---

[3] Available at: www.who.int/reproductivehealth/topics/maternal_perinatal/augmentation-labour

cutting applicability issues as informed by the limits of the prioritized recommendation questions. These principles, in addition to the strategies for implementation, monitoring and evaluation presented later in the document, are expected to guide end-users in the process of adapting and implementing the guideline in a range of contexts and settings.

- Application of the recommendations should be based on consideration of the general condition of the woman and her baby, her wishes and preferences, and respect for her dignity and autonomy.
- Augmentation of labour should be performed only when there is a clear medical indication and the expected benefits outweigh the potential harms.
- Women undergoing augmentation of labour, particularly with oxytocin, should not be left unattended.
- Augmentation of labour with oxytocin is appropriate and should only be performed after conducting clinical assessment to exclude cephalopelvic disproportion. This principle is relevant for all women but is even more crucial for multiparous women.
- As the evidence for these recommendations was largely informed by studies conducted among women with pregnancies in cephalic presentation and unscarred uterus, they should not be applied to women with abnormal fetal presentation (including breech) or scarred uterus.
- Augmentation of labour should be performed with caution as the procedure carries the risk of uterine hyperstimulation, with the potential consequences of fetal distress and uterine rupture.
- Wherever augmentation of labour is performed, facilities should be available to closely and regularly monitor fetal heart rate and uterine contraction pattern.
- Augmentation of labour should be carried out in facilities where there is capacity to manage its potential outcomes, including adverse effects and failure to achieve spontaneous vaginal birth.

3.2 Definition of delay in the first stage of labour

The GDG acknowledged that there are variable definitions of what constitutes delay in the progress of the first stage of labour, but it is most often dependent on the rate of cervical dilatation. A cervical dilatation rate of less than 0.5 cm to 1 cm per hour during the active phase (i.e. the period of labour associated with dilatation of the cervix from approximately 3–4 cm to 10 cm) is commonly considered to be slow progress of labour, with the trigger for intervention stipulated at a variable period following such deviation. While it is widely acknowledged that labour tends to be faster among multiparous compared to nulliparous women, the same criteria often apply for identification of delay in both groups in clinical practice.

In recognition of a lack of universal consensus on the definition of delay in labour and the variable definitions used in the research that formed the evidence base for these recommendations, the GDG agreed that adopting a specific definition for delayed labour might threaten the applicability of the guideline across all settings. Rather, the group emphasized that the standard that is followed should allow individual institutions or clinicians adequate time for clinical assessment and interventions (including referral) such that the desired benefits for both mother and baby can be achieved.

3.3 Evidence and recommendations

The WHO technical consultation adopted 20 recommendations covering prioritized questions related to the diagnosis, prevention and treatment of delay in the progress of the first stage of labour, and supportive care for women undergoing labour augmentation. The diagnosis and prevention aspects of the recommendations focus on methods to assess the progress of labour (see Recommendations Nos. 1 and 2) and intrapartum interventions usually performed to prevent delay in labour and thus avoid the use of labour augmentation (see Recommendations Nos. 3 to 13). The recommendations regarding treatment of delay in labour are specific to the pharmacological and nonpharmacological methods of augmenting labour (see Recommendations Nos. 14 to 19). The recommendation on care during augmentation applies to methods of assessing maternal uterine response to the labour augmentation process (see Recommendation No. 20). The quality of the supporting evidence (very low, low, moderate or high) and the strength of each recommendation (strong or weak) are indicated. To ensure that each recommendation is correctly understood and used appropriately in practice, additional remarks reflecting the summary of the discussion by the GDG are noted for each recommendation, where necessary. While the interventions reviewed mostly relate to prevention and management of delay in the first stage of labour, the GDG also considered other key elements of women-centred care in its recommendations.

3.3.1 Diagnosis of delay in the first stage of labour

Recommendation No. 1: Active phase partograph with a four-hour action line is recommended for monitoring the progress of labour. (Strong recommendation, very low quality of evidence)

Remarks

- The GDG acknowledged the low quality of the supporting evidence but noted that many units in both high- and low-income settings currently use the partograph and, although no clinical benefits in health outcomes were reported in the RCTs, it is a useful tool for providing a pictorial overview of progress, clinical audit, training of health workers and facilitating the transfer of care. These considerations, in addition to the low resource implication of the intervention led the GDG to make a strong recommendation in favour of the partograph.

- The potential benefits of introducing the use of a partograph may be more apparent in under-resourced clinical settings where a standard protocol for labour management is either not used or is inconsistently used. However, the benefits of using the partograph can only be maximized when accompanied by adherence to a standard labour management protocol.

- Considering the variability among women with regard to rates of progress during labour, the GDG placed its emphasis on reducing the likelihood of unnecessary interventions and therefore chose to recommend the four-hour action line partograph rather than those with earlier action lines.

Evidence summary: Partograph for monitoring the progress of labour (EB Tables 1a–1n)*

- Evidence on the use of a partograph as a monitoring tool to identify when intervention becomes indicated during labour was extracted from a Cochrane systematic review of six RCTs (> 7000 women) *(15)*. The review examined seven different comparisons, but few data could be pooled in meta-analysis.

Partograph versus no partograph

- Two trials conducted in Canada and Mexico involving a total of 1590 women compared partograph with no partograph.

- In one trial, there were no significant differences in the mean duration (MD) of the first (MD 0.8 hrs, 95% CI −0.06 to 1.66) or second (MD 0 hrs, 95% CI −0.21 to 0.21) stages of labour.

- Overall, there was no significant difference in the frequency of caesarean section (RR 0.64, 95% CI 0.24 to 1.70), although findings in the two trials were not consistent. In the Canadian trial, there was no significant difference between groups (RR 1.03, 95% CI 0.82 to 1.28; 1156 women), whereas significantly fewer women in the partograph group had caesarean section in the Mexican trial (RR 0.38, 95% CI 0.24 to 0.61; 434 women). The Mexican trial, however, was at high risk of bias due to poor allocation concealment.

- There were no significant differences between groups for the other critical or important maternal and infant outcomes reported: use of epidural (RR 1.01, 95% CI 0.98 to 1.05); oxytocin augmentation (RR 1.02, 95% CI 0.95 to 1.1); instrumental vaginal birth (RR 1.00, 95% CI 0.85 to 1.17); artificial rupture of the membranes (RR 0.99, 95% CI 0.88 to 1.11); low Apgar score at five minutes (RR 0.77, 95% CI 0.29 to 2.06); and admission to special care nursery (RR 0.94, 95% CI 0.51 to 1.75).

continued...

---

* These and all EB tables are presented in the Evidence base document, available at: www.who.int/reproductivehealth/topics/maternal_perinatal/augmentation-labour

> **Recommendation No. 1:** Active phase partograph with a four-hour action line is recommended for monitoring the progress of labour. (Strong recommendation, very low quality of evidence)

Partograph with an alert line only versus one with both alert and action lines

- A trial involving 694 women in South Africa compared a partograph with an alert line only with one with both alert and action lines. Women in the alert line only group received what was described as "aggressive" labour management with two-hourly vaginal examinations and oxytocin augmentation once the alert line was crossed. Women in the other group received expectant management with four-hourly vaginal examinations and oxytocin augmentation when the action line (four hrs to the right of the alert line) was crossed. It was unclear whether the findings reflected the use of different types of partograph or other features of labour management.

- Women in the alert line only group were significantly less likely to have caesarean section (RR 0.68, 95% CI 0.50 to 0.93). Rates of oxytocin augmentation (RR 0.81, 95% CI 0.62 to 1.05) and instrumental vaginal birth (RR 0.87, 95% CI 0.66 to 1.15) were similar between the groups.

- There were insufficient events to detect differences in terms of the infant outcomes reported: perinatal death (RR 7.12, 95% CI 0.37 to 137.36) and low Apgar score at five minutes (RR 7.12, 95% CI 0.37 to 137.36).

Partograph with two-hour versus four-hour action lines

- Two trials conducted in the United Kingdom compared partographs with two-hour versus four-hour action lines.

- There were no significant differences between the comparison groups for reported critical or important maternal outcomes: caesarean section for all indications (RR 1.06, 95% CI 0.85 to 1.32); caesarean section for fetal distress (RR 1.30, 95% CI 0.86 to 1.96); caesarean section for delay in labour (RR 0.98, 95% CI 0.77 to 1.25); use of epidural (RR 1.04, 95% CI 0.95 to 1.14); instrumental vaginal (RR 0.91, 95% CI 0.80 to 1.03); and postpartum haemorrhage (PPH) (RR 1.07, 95% CI 0.90 to 1.26).

- There was a modest increase in the number of women receiving oxytocin augmentation in the two-hour partograph group (RR 1.14, 95% CI 1.05 to 1.22; two trials, 3601 women).

- There were no significant differences in infant outcomes reported: Apgar score < 7 at five minutes (RR 0.82, 95% CI 0.5 to 1.35); cord pH < 7.1 (RR 0.73, 95% CI 0.44 to 1.22); and admission to special care nursery (RR 0.78, 95% CI 0.46 to 1.31).

Partograph with two-hour versus three-hour action lines

- One trial in the United Kingdom compared partograph with two-hour versus three-hour action lines. There were no statistically significant differences between these partograph designs for any of the maternal or infant outcomes reported.

- Maternal outcomes: caesarean section for all indications (RR 0.78, 95% CI 0.51 to 1.18); caesarean section for fetal distress (RR 0.96, 95% CI 0.44 to 2.1); caesarean section for delay in labour (RR 0.71, 95% CI 0.42 to 1.19); use of epidural (RR 1.16, 95% CI 0.94 to 1.44); oxytocin augmentation (RR 1.02, 95% CI 0.85 to 1.21); instrumental vaginal birth (RR 0.93, 95% CI 0.69 to 1.26); and PPH (RR 0.96, 95% CI 0.63 to 1.45).

- Infant outcomes: Apgar score < 7 at five minutes (RR 1.44, 95% CI 0.41 to 5.05); cord pH < 7.1 (RR 0.38, 95% CI 0.07 to 1.96); and admission to special care nursery (RR 3.83, 95% CI 0.43 to 34.12). Other infant outcomes were not reported.

continued...

Recommendation No. 1: Active phase partograph with a four-hour action line is recommended for monitoring the progress of labour. (Strong recommendation, very low quality of evidence)

Partograph with three-hour versus four-hour action lines

- One trial in the United Kingdom compared partographs with three-hour versus four-hour action lines. There were no statistically significant differences between these partograph designs for most of the maternal and infant outcomes reported.

- The rates of caesarean section for fetal distress or for delay in labour in the two groups were not significantly different (RR 1.77, 95% CI 0.70 to 4.42, and RR 1.68, 95% CI 0.97 to 2.91, respectively). However, in the trial (613 women), overall rate of caesarean section was higher in the three-hour compared with the four-hour action line group (RR 1.70, 95% CI 1.07 to 2.70). Results for other maternal outcomes did not identify statistically significant differences between women cared for using the two partograph designs: PPH (blood loss > 500 ml) (RR 1.03, 95% CI 0.68 to 1.56); use of epidural (RR 1.01, 95% CI 0.80 to 1.27); oxytocin augmentation (RR 1.09, 95% CI 0.91 to 1.30); and instrumental vaginal birth (RR 0.96, 95% CI 0.72 to 1.28).

- There were no significant differences between any of the infant outcomes reported: low Apgar score at five minutes (RR 0.82, 95% CI 0.22 to 3.04); cord pH < 7.1 (RR 2.57, 95% CI 0.5 to 13.17); and admission to special care nursery (RR 0.51, 95% CI 0.05 to 5.65).

Partograph prompting early versus later intervention

- The trial conducted in South Africa was pooled with the two trials from the United Kingdom trials in a comparison examining partograph designs prompting earlier versus later intervention. Overall, there were no significant differences between earlier and later intervention for the outcomes reported: caesarean section (RR 0.94, 95% CI 0.67 to 1.31), and instrumental birth (RR 0.9, 95% CI 0.8 to 1.02).

Partograph with latent phase versus partograph without latent phase

- One trial conducted in India with data for 743 women compared a partograph design with a latent phase with one without a latent phase.

- Women cared for using a partograph with a latent phase were more likely to have caesarean section for all indications (RR 2.45, 95% CI 1.72 to 3.50) and specifically for fetal distress (RR 4.87, 95% CI 2.83 to 8.37). The difference between the groups in rates of caesarean section for delay was not statistically significant (RR 1.35, 95% CI 0.59 to 3.08).

- The partograph with a latent phase was also associated with increased use of oxytocin augmentation (RR 2.18, 95% CI 1.67 to 2.83). There was no difference between the groups in the frequencies of instrumental vaginal birth (RR 1.04, 95% CI 0.61 to 1.77).

- No significant difference was observed for low Apgar scores at five minutes (RR 0.75, 95% CI 0.21 to 2.63), but infants in the latent phase partograph group were more likely to be admitted to special care nursery (RR 1.84, 95% CI 1.29 to 2.63). Other maternal and neonatal outcomes were not reported.

Overall quality of evidence

- Overall, the quality of the evidence for most outcomes was graded as very low.

Recommendation No. 2: Digital vaginal examination at intervals of four hours is recommended for routine assessment and identification of delay in active labour. (Weak recommendation, very low quality of evidence)

Remarks

- The specified time interval reflects the period between the alert and action lines of the partograph (see Recommendation No. 1) and further reinforces the need to allow time to confirm the diagnosis of delay in labour before instituting any intervention.

- The GDG acknowledged that vaginal examination at more frequent intervals might be indicated the condition of the mother or the baby. In any case, priority must be given to the woman's wishes and preferences and to minimizing the total number of vaginal examinations.

- Rectal examination can be more uncomfortable for women and should not be performed.

Evidence summary: Routine vaginal examination for assessing the progress of labour (EB Tables 2a–2c)

- Evidence was extracted from a Cochrane systematic review of two trials *(16)*, each examining a different comparison. One trial conducted in Ireland in 307 women with ruptured membranes compared routine vaginal examinations (one–two hourly) with rectal examinations to assess progress in labour. A trial in the United Kingdom compared two-hourly with four-hourly vaginal examinations in nulliparous women in labour (in this trial 150 women were randomized but 109 women were included in the analysis).

Vaginal versus rectal examinations in labour: maternal and infant outcomes

- The trial conducted in Ireland (307 women) showed that there were no significant differences between women undergoing vaginal versus rectal examinations with respect to maternal outcomes: caesarean section (RR 0.33, 95% CI 0.03 to 3.15); spontaneous vaginal birth (RR 0.98, 95% CI 0.9 to 1.06); operative vaginal birth (RR 1.38, 95% CI 0.70 to 2.71); and augmentation of labour (RR 1.03, 95% CI 0.63 to 1.68). There was also no significant difference between the groups in the rate of infection (not defined) (RR 0.50, 95% CI 0.22 to 1.13).

- Women were less likely to report that vaginal examinations in labour were uncomfortable compared with rectal ones (RR 0.42, 95% CI 0.25 to 0.70).

- For infant outcomes, there were no significant differences between the groups for any of the outcomes reported, and for most outcomes the estimates were based on very low event rates: perinatal mortality (RR 0.99, 95% CI 0.06 to 15.74); neonatal infection requiring antibiotics (RR 0.33, 95% CI 0.01 to 8.07); other neonatal infection (RR 0.99, 95% CI 0.14 to 6.96); and admission to neonatal intensive care unit (NICU) (RR 1.32, 95% CI 0.47 to 3.73).

Two-hourly versus four-hourly vaginal examinations in labour: maternal and infant outcomes

- In the trial in the United Kingdom comparing two-hourly versus four-hourly vaginal examinations to assess progress in labour there were no significant differences between the groups for any of the maternal outcomes reported: length of labour (MD –6.00 min, 95% CI –88.7 to 76.7); caesarean section (RR 0.77, 95% CI 0.36 to 1.64; operative vaginal birth (RR 1.44, 95% CI 0.66 to 3.17); use of epidural for pain relief (RR 0.77, 95% CI 0.39 to 1.55); and use of labour augmentation for slow progress (RR 1.03, 95% CI 0.64 to 1.67).

- No infant outcomes were reported.

Overall quality of evidence

- The overall quality of the evidence was graded as very low.

3.3.2 Prevention of delay in the first stage of labour

Recommendation No. 3: A package of care for active management of labour for prevention of delay in labour is not recommended. (Weak recommendation, low quality of evidence)

Remarks

- The GDG agreed that this package of interventions has potential benefits in terms of reducing the duration of labour and possibly caesarean section rate. However, the group did not support its recommendation as it considered the approach to be highly prescriptive and interventional and one that could undermine women's rights, choices and autonomy as recipients of care. In addition, the intervention is considered to be a complex package that exerts considerable demands on health resources, which may not be feasible in many settings. The GDG chose not to recommend the package because the reported clinical benefits do not clearly outweigh these other considerations.

- The GDG also noted that continuous one-to-one care is the only component of the package that has been shown to be beneficial, and is probably the component responsible for the benefits attributed to the package. Continuous support during labour as a separate intervention is recommended in this guideline (see Recommendation No. 12)

Evidence summary: Package of care for active management of labour for prevention of delay in the first stage of labour (EB Tables 3a–3b)

- Evidence on packages of care for the active management of labour compared with routine care was extracted from a Cochrane systematic review of seven trials (> 5000 women) *(6)*.

- The trials were conducted in high-, middle- and low-income countries: three in the United States of America (USA) and one each in Belgium, New Zealand, Thailand and Nigeria.

- All but one of the trials recruited women in early spontaneous labour. To be included in the review, the predefined package of care in labour had to be clearly described in trial reports and care had to include more than two, or all of the key elements described traditionally as "active management of labour": early routine amniotomy and augmentation with oxytocin; strict criteria for the diagnosis of labour, abnormal progress in labour and fetal compromise; continual presence of a midwife/nurse during labour; peer review of assisted deliveries and progress of labour plotted using a graph. The comparative care in the included trials was also clearly described.

- Most of the included trials used higher starting and increment oxytocin doses for women receiving the package of care for active management of labour compared to those receiving usual care.

Package of care for active management in labour versus routine care: maternal outcomes

- None of the trials reported maternal mortality.

- There was a statistically significant reduction in the duration of labour for women in the active management of labour group (MD –1.27 hrs, 95% CI –2.19 to –0.36; four trials, 2431 women). The direction of the effect was consistent in all trials, with women in the intervention group having shorter labour; however, the size of the mean reduction varied considerably in different trials from between a few minutes to up to two hours.

- There was a significant reduction in the length of the first stage of labour (MD –1.56, 95% CI –2.17 to –0.96; four trials, 2431 women). The length of the second stage of labour was very similar in the two groups (MD –0.02, 95% CI –0.06 to 0.02; five trials, 2737 women).

- There was no significant difference in the frequencies of PPH (blood loss > 500 ml) between the comparison groups (RR 0.93, 95% CI 0.67 to 1.31; three trials, 1504 women).

continued...

> **Recommendation No. 3:** A package of care for active management of labour for prevention of delay in labour is not recommended. (Weak recommendation, low quality of evidence)

Package of care for active management in labour versus routine care: maternal outcomes (continued)

- For caesarean section, the observed difference between groups was not statistically significant, although there was a trend towards a modest reduction in caesarean section in the active management group (RR 0.88, 95% CI 0.77 to 1.01; seven trials, 5390 women). More than 40% of the weight in this analysis was due to a trial that recruited women early in the third trimester and by labour more than a third of them were no longer eligible. If data for women who were still eligible at the time of labour are included, the pooled effect size is increased, and the difference between the groups is statistically significant, favouring active management (RR 0.82, 95% CI 0.69 to 0.97; seven trials, 4738 women). If data from this trial are excluded altogether the difference between groups remains significant (RR 0.77, 95% CI 0.63 to 0.94; six trials, 3475 women).

- The frequency of prolonged labour (defined as > 12 hrs) was considerably reduced in the active management group (RR 0.47, 95% CI 0.32 to 0.69; six trials, 3242 women).

- There were no clear differences between the groups for rates of assisted vaginal birth (RR 0.99, 95% CI 0.87 to 1.14) or epidural analgesia (RR 1.06, 95% CI 0.98 to 1.14).

- There was no significant difference between the groups for maternal infection (various definitions) (RR 1.14, 95% CI 0.65 to 1.98).

- Maternal satisfaction with experience during labour was very similar in both groups (RR 1.04, 95% CI 0.94 to 1.15).

Package of care for active management in labour versus routine care: infant outcomes

- Few infant outcomes were reported in this review. There were no statistically significant differences in admission to NICU (RR 0.92, 95% CI 0.59 to 1.43), Apgar score < 7 at five minutes (RR 1.12, 95% CI 0.76 to 1.64) or meconium staining (RR 0.93, 95% CI 0.7 to 1.24).

Overall quality of evidence

- Overall, the quality of the evidence was graded as low.

- Evidence relating to the use of amniotomy alone, oxytocin alone or early amniotomy with early oxytocin is presented separately in this document.

Recommendation No. 4: The use of early amniotomy with early oxytocin augmentation for prevention of delay in labour is not recommended. (Weak recommendation, very low quality of evidence)

Remarks

- The GDG noted that the variable reduction in the first stage of labour itself does not justify the interventions given that no substantive differences were found in other important clinical outcomes.

- The GDG noted the substantial overlap between this intervention and the components of active management of labour and considered it as equally highly prescriptive and interventional. Like the package of active management of labour (see Recommendation No. 3), the group placed much emphasis on its potential to undermine women's rights, choices and autonomy as recipients of care, and therefore did not recommended the intervention. Additionally, the intervention is not considered feasible in many settings, as it requires considerable health-care resources to implement.

Evidence summary: Early amniotomy and early oxytocin for prevention of delay in the first stage of labour (EB Tables 4a–4c)

- Evidence on the use of early amniotomy and early oxytocin compared with routine care for preventing delay in labour was extracted from a Cochrane systematic review of 11 RCTs (> 7000 women) *(17)*.

- Trials were conducted in both high- and low-resource settings: four in the USA, and one each in Belgium, Chile, France, India, New Zealand, Nigeria, and Thailand.

- Women in early spontaneous labour with detected slow progress were allocated to early amniotomy and oxytocin versus usual care. Four of the trials included in the review included the use of early amniotomy and early oxytocin as part of a package of care for the active management of labour (which included strict diagnosis of labour, regular vaginal examinations to assess progress and one-to-one care). A sensitivity analysis was conducted excluding these trials from the main analysis to examine the impact on results.

Early amniotomy and early oxytocin for the prevention of delay: maternal outcomes

- Only one trial reported on maternal mortality; there were no maternal deaths in either group.

- Overall, trials showed a statistically significant reduction in the total duration of labour (from admission) for women in the intervention group (MD −1.11 hrs, 95% CI −1.82 to −0.41; seven trials, 4675 women). The direction of effect was consistent in all trials, with women in the intervention group having shorter labour; however, the size of the mean reduction varied considerably in different trials ranging from a few minutes to more than two hours. The difference between groups remained significant in the sensitivity analysis (excluding trials that used early amniotomy and oxytocin as part of active management of labour) (MD −0.81 hrs, 95% CI −1.36 to −0.25; five trials, 3822 women).

- There was a significant reduction in the length of the first stage of labour for women in the intervention group in the overall analysis (MD −1.57 hrs, 95% CI −2.15 to −1.00; four trials, 4675 women) and in the sensitivity analysis (MD −1.27 hrs, 95% CI −2.08 to −0.47; two trials, 1578 women).

- Overall, there was a modest reduction in the number of women in the intervention group undergoing caesarean section for any indication (RR 0.87, 95% CI 0.77 to 0.99; 11 trials, 7753 women). The difference between the groups for caesarean section was not significant in the sensitivity analysis, but there was a trend towards more women in the intervention group being less likely to undergo caesarean section (RR 0.84, 95% CI 0.70 to 1.01; seven trials, 4885 women).

- Maternal satisfaction with experience during childbirth was similar between comparison groups (RR 1.02, 95% CI 0.99 to 1.04; two trials, 2436 women).

continued...

> **Recommendation No. 4: The use of early amniotomy with early oxytocin augmentation for prevention of delay in labour is not recommended. (Weak recommendation, very low quality of evidence)**
>
> *Early amniotomy and early oxytocin for the prevention of delay: maternal outcomes (continued)*
>
> - Overall, there were no significant difference between groups for hyperstimulation of labour (RR 1.37, 95% CI 0.76 to 2.46; two trials, 853 women), PPH (blood loss > 500 ml) (RR 0.83, 95% CI 0.65 to 1.08; four trials, 2674 women), maternal blood transfusion (RR 1.84, 95% CI 0.32 to 10.48; three trials, 2977 women) or postpartum fever or infection (RR 0.88, 95% CI 0.66 to 1.16; five trials, 2824 women). Sensitivity analyses (excluding the active management of labour trials) showed that the occurrences of PPH, maternal blood transfusion and postpartum infection or fever were also not significantly different between the intervention and control groups. Hyperstimulation of labour was not reported in the trials included in the sensitivity analysis.
>
> *Early amniotomy and early oxytocin for the prevention of delay: infant outcomes*
>
> - For neonatal outcomes, there were no statistically significant differences in serious neonatal morbidity: seizure/neurological abnormalities (RR 0.83, 95% CI 0.25 to 2.71; two trials, 2666 women); abnormal arterial cord pH (acidosis) (RR 1.11, 95% CI 0.61 to 2.02; three trials, 1416 women); jaundice or hyperbilirubinaemia (RR 1.10, 95% CI 0.68 to 1.77; two trials, 2219 women); admission to NICU (RR 1.13, 95% CI 0.91 to 1.41; six trials, 4479 women); and Apgar score < 7 at five minutes (RR 1.10, 95% CI 0.77 to 1.55; six trials, 4479 women). The sensitivity analysis showed similar observations for the above-listed infant outcomes.
>
> *Overall quality of evidence*
>
> - Overall, the quality of the evidence was graded very low.
>
> - Evidence relating to the use of amniotomy alone, oxytocin alone and both amniotomy and oxytocin as part of a package of care for active management of labour is presented separately.

Recommendation No. 5: The use of oxytocin for prevention of delay in labour in women receiving epidural analgesia is not recommended. (Weak recommendation, low quality of evidence)
Remarks
• Augmentation with oxytocin should be performed when indicated as treatment of confirmed delay of labour progress in women receiving epidural analgesia.
Evidence summary: Oxytocin for prevention of delay in labour in women under epidural analgesia (EB Tables 5a–5b)

- Evidence relating to the routine use of oxytocin for improving outcomes for women undergoing epidural analgesia in labour was extracted from a Cochrane systematic review of two trials (319 women) comparing oxytocin augmentation with placebo (saline) for women undergoing epidural analgesia who otherwise would have been managed expectantly *(18)*. Both trials were carried out in the United Kingdom and only included nulliparous women in spontaneous labour. One of the trials randomized 226 women at full cervical dilatation while the other recruited 93 women at six cm or less cervical dilatation.

- There were no statistically significant differences between comparison groups for any of the critical or important outcomes reported.

Oxytocin versus placebo for women under epidural analgesia: maternal outcomes

- No significant differences were observed between the groups in the incidence of PPH (RR 0.96, 95% CI 0.58 to 1.59), overall caesarean section rate (RR 0.95, 95% CI 0.42 to 2.12), instrumental vaginal birth (RR 0.88, 95% CI 0.72 to 1.08) or uterine hyperstimulation (RR 1.32, 95% CI 0.97 to 1.8).

Oxytocin versus placebo for women under epidural analgesia: infant outcomes

- Few neonatal outcomes were reported. Compared to women receiving placebo, those who received oxytocin had similar observations for infants with low Apgar scores at five minutes (RR 3.06, 95% CI 0.13 to 73.33), and admission to NICU (RR 1.07, 95% CI 0.29 to 3.93), although data were very sparse for both of these outcomes.

Overall quality of evidence

- The overall quality of the evidence was graded as low.

- Evidence on the use of oxytocin for women with dystocia, or as part of a package of care for the active management of labour is presented separately.

> **Recommendation No. 6:** The use of amniotomy alone for prevention of delay in labour is not recommended. (Weak recommendation, very low quality of evidence)

Remarks

- The GDG noted that in spite of the common use of amniotomy for prevention of labour delay in clinical practice there is no clear evidence that the potential benefits outweigh harms. Although the GDG acknowledged the simplicity of performing the procedure and its feasibility in many settings, they chose not to recommend the intervention in favour of avoiding unnecessary discomfort to the woman and the concept of reducing medicalization of childbirth.

- As early amniotomy may increase the risk of perinatal HIV transmission, this recommendation could be strengthened in settings where HIV infection is prevalent and women may present in labour with unknown HIV status.

Evidence summary: The use of routine amniotomy (alone) for prevention of delay in the first stage of labour (EB Tables 6a–6b)

- Evidence related to the use of amniotomy as a single intervention to prevent delay in the first stage of labour was drawn from a Cochrane systematic review of 14 RCTs (> 5000 women) comparing routine amniotomy versus intention to preserve amniotic membranes *(19)*.

- Women were recruited in early labour and were progressing normally at the point of randomization. Results were reported overall, and for primiparous and multiparous women separately.

- Trials were predominantly conducted in high-resource settings (11 trials in Europe, Canada and the USA, and one trial each in Iran, Nigeria and the Palestinian West Bank).

Routine amniotomy versus intention to preserve amniotic membranes (no routine amniotomy): maternal outcomes

- Overall, there was no significant reduction in the length of the first stage (MD −20.43 min, 95% CI −95.93 to 55.06; five trials, 1127 women) or the second stage (MD −1.33 min, 95% CI −2.92 to 0.26; eight trials, 1927 women) of labour. However, there was a statistically significant but modest reduction in the length of the second stage of labour for primiparous women (MD −5.43 min, 95% CI −9.98 to −0.89; seven trials, 653 women).

- For caesarean section, the observed difference between the groups was not statistically significant, but there was a trend towards an increased risk in the amniotomy group (RR 1.27, 95% CI 0.99 to 1.63; nine trials, 5021 women). The only trial that reported caesarean section by indication showed no difference between the groups: caesarean section for fetal distress (RR 3.21, 95% CI 0.66 to 15.6); caesarean section for prolonged labour (RR 0.45, 95% CI 0.07 to 3.03).

- A significantly lower risk of "dysfunctional labour" was reported for women in the routine amniotomy group (RR 0.60, 95% CI 0.44 to 0.82; three trials, 1695 women).

- Three trials (1740 women) reported maternal mortality. There was one maternal death recorded and no difference was observed between the groups.

- In three trials (2150 women), there was no observed difference in the rates of maternal infection (RR 0.88, 95% CI 0.43 to 1.82). None of the trials in the review reported other indicators of serious maternal morbidity.

- No significant difference was observed in the incidence of PPH (blood loss > 500 ml) (RR 0.46, 95% CI 0.14 to 1.50; two trials, 1822 women).

- Two trials reported very low and similar incidence of cord prolapse in both groups.

continued...

> **Recommendation No. 6: The use of amniotomy alone for prevention of delay in labour is not recommended.**
> **(Weak recommendation, very low quality of evidence)**
>
> *Routine amniotomy versus intention to preserve amniotic membranes (no routine amniotomy): infant outcomes*
>
> - Overall, there was a paucity of data for critical and important neonatal outcomes and no differences were observed in any of those reported.
>
> - No significant differences were observed between the groups for perinatal death (RR 3.01, 95% CI 0.12 to 73.59; eight trials) or indicators of neonatal morbidity: seizures (RR 0.88, 95% CI 0.15 to 5.35; five trials); intracranial haemorrhage (no estimable data); respiratory distress syndrome (RR 0.20, 95% CI 0.01 to 4.16; two trials); meconium aspiration syndrome (RR 3.06, 95% CI 0.83 to 11.27; two trials); cephalohaematoma (RR 1.52, 95% CI 0.81 to 2.83; three trials); fracture (RR 3.01, 95% CI 0.31 to 28.80; one trial); jaundice (RR 0.90, 95% CI 0.76 to 1.06; five trials); and admission to NICU (RR 1.08, 95% CI 0.77 to 1.50; five trials).
>
> - There was no observed difference between groups for acidosis (defined as cord blood arterial pH < 7.2) (RR 1.18, 95% CI 0.8 to 1.73; two trials), although a trend towards a reduction in Apgar score < 7 at five minutes was reported for neonates in the routine amniotomy group (RR 0.53, 95% CI 0.28 to 1.00; six trials, 3598 women).
>
> *Overall quality of evidence*
>
> - Overall, the quality of the evidence was graded as very low.
>
> - Evidence relating to the use of amniotomy with early oxytocin, and the use of amniotomy and oxytocin as part of a package of care involving other interventions is presented separately.

> **Recommendation No. 7:** The use of antispasmodic agents for prevention of delay in labour is not recommended. (Weak recommendation, very low quality of evidence)

Remarks

- The GDG noted that the available data were too heterogeneous with respect to the participants and interventions to permit wide applicability of the results. The shortening in the length of the first stage of labour by one hour was considered clinically inconsequential, as it did not translate to improvement in the other critical maternal or infant outcomes. The GDG placed a high value on safety issues, which were poorly reported, and chose not to recommend the practice until new information demonstrating clinical benefits with minimal risks becomes available.

- The GDG considers the use of antispasmodic agents for treatment of delay in labour as a research priority.

> **Evidence summary: Antispasmodics for prevention of delay in labour (EB Tables 7a–7b)**

- Evidence on the use of antispasmodics compared with placebo or no medication for shortening the duration of labour was drawn from a Cochrane systematic review of 21 RCTs (3286 women) *(20)*.

- The review included heterogeneous groups of participants, interventions and outcomes. Ten trials included only primigravid women, one only multigravid women, nine included both and one did not specify the gravidity of participants.

- One trial included only women with induction of labour, two included both women following induction or in spontaneous labour, 13 trials only included participants in spontaneous labour, and five trials did not specify whether participants were in spontaneous or induced labour.

- Antispasmodics with musculotropic effects (drotaverine hydrochloride, rociverine and camylofin dihydrochloride) and those with neurotropic effects (valethamate bromide and hyoscine butyl-bromide) were reported separately. Most of the trials included in the review (14) used antispasmodics followed by a protocol of active management of labour, which included amniotomy, augmentation with oxytocin, or both, and only two trials avoided amniotomy and oxytocin augmentation, while five trials did not mention amniotomy or oxytocin. Antispasmodic drugs were administered intravenously, intramuscularly or per rectum.

- All but one of the trials recruited women with low-risk pregnancies.

- Evidence related to the duration of labour and the rate of cervical dilatation was extracted from trials that excluded data for women whose final mode of delivery was caesarean section.

- The 21 trials were conducted in India (nine trials), Iran (three), Saudi Arabia (two), Turkey (two) and Italy, Nepal, Kenya, Jamaica and the USA (one each).

Antispasmodics versus control: maternal outcomes

- No trials reported on maternal mortality.

- Using findings from trials that excluded data for women who had caesarean section when estimating mean duration of labour, there was a significant reduction in the duration of the first stage of labour (MD −59.10 min, 95% CI −95.81 to −22.38; seven trials, 1051 women) but no significant reduction in the length of the second stage of labour (MD 0.51 min, 95% CI −3.04 to 4.06; six trials, 753 women). There was a significant reduction in the total duration of labour for vaginal births in the antispasmodic group (MD −102.60 min, 95% CI −164.12 to −41.08; three trials, 392 women). This reduction was significant overall, and for neurotropic agents (MD −80.78 min, 95% CI −153.81 to −7.75; three trials, 244 women), but did not reach statistical significance for musculotropic agents (MD −138.21 min, 95% CI −291.51 to 15.09; two trials, 148 women).

- The rate of cervical dilatation for vaginal births was significantly faster with antispasmodics compared with control (MD 0.67 cm/hr, 95% CI 0.39 to 0.95; four trials, 553 women).

continued...

> **Recommendation No. 7:** The use of antispasmodic agents for prevention of delay in labour is not recommended. (Weak recommendation, very low quality of evidence)
>
> *Antispasmodics versus control: maternal outcomes (continued)*
> - The rate of caesarean section or instrumental vaginal birth was not reported in the review. However, no significant difference was observed in the rate of normal vertex deliveries between antispasmodics and control (RR 1.02, 95% CI 1.00 to 1.05; 16 trials, 2319 women).
> - With respect to adverse events, no significant differences were observed in the incidence of cervical laceration between antispasmodics and control (RR 0.79, 95% CI 0.20 to 3.12), although few trials addressed this outcome and the number of events was small.
> - Overall, there was no difference observed in the incidence of PPH (blood loss > 500 ml) (RR 2.46 95% CI 0.20 to 30.17), but one trial (100 women) showed a marginal increase in PPH risk for drotaverine hydrochloride, a musculotropic agent (RR 9.00, 95% CI 1.18 to 68.42). There was no significant difference in PPH observed between neurotropic agents and the control group (RR 0.75, 95% CI 0.13 to 4.26; one trial).
> - The incidence of maternal tachycardia was significantly higher for antispasmodic agents compared with control (RR 4.54, 95% CI 2.53 to 8.16). This effect was significantly different for neurotropic agents whereas it was similar between comparison groups for musculotropic agents. Similar effects were observed for mouth dryness and flushing of the face.
> - There were no significant differences between antispasmodic agents and control in the occurrence of maternal adverse events such as headache, nausea, vomiting, dizziness and giddiness.
>
> *Antispasmodics versus control: infant outcomes*
> - No trials reported data for perinatal death.
> - Overall, there were no significant differences between groups for admission to NICU (RR 0.84, 95% CI 0.34 to 2.05).
> - One trial reported fetal distress, with no significant difference between comparison groups (RR 0.50, 95% CI 0.10 to 2.61).
> - One trial reported fetal bradycardia, with no significant difference between groups (RR 0.67, 95% CI 0.12 to 3.86).
> - Two trials reported fetal tachycardia for neurotropic agents, with no significant difference between groups (RR 3.40, 95% CI 0.85 to 13.67).
> - One trial reported meconium-stained liquor. However it was a small sample, there were few events, and the difference was not significant (RR 2.04, 95% CI 0.54 to 7.73).
>
> *Overall quality of evidence*
> - Overall, the quality of the evidence was graded as very low.

> **Recommendation No. 8: Pain relief for preventing delay and reducing the use of augmentation in labour is not recommended. (Weak recommendation, very low quality of evidence)**

Remarks

- The GDG noted that there is no clear evidence to suggest that any form of pain relief is associated with reduction in labour duration and frequency of labour augmentation.

- The GDG acknowledged that pain relief may not necessarily reduce the need for labour augmentation but it has other substantial benefits that make it an essential component of good intrapartum care.

Evidence summary: Effect of pain relief on duration of labour and oxytocin augmentation (EB Tables 8a–8n)

- Evidence related to the effects of pain relief on the duration of labour and use of oxytocin for augmentation was extracted from 11 Cochrane systematic reviews *(21–31)*. Several other systematic reviews examining pain relief in labour (e.g. reviews on inhaled analgesia or intravenous and intramuscular opioids) did not include these outcomes, and data from these reviews were not included.

Epidural versus nonepidural analgesia in labour

- Data were extracted from 17 trials involving more than 5000 women *(21)*. Eight trials were conducted in the USA, two in the United Kingdom, and one each in Sweden, Denmark, China, Taiwan, India, Mexico and Iran.

- There was no significant difference in the duration of the first stage of labour (MD 18.51 min, 95% CI −12.91 to 49.92). The second stage of labour appeared significantly shorter in women in the control group (no epidural) although there was considerable variation in the size and direction of effect among the different trials (MD 13.66 min, 95% CI 6.67 to 20.66; 13 trials, > 4000 women.

- Women receiving epidural were more likely to require labour augmentation, although again the size and direction of the effect was not consistent (RR 1.19, 95% CI 1.03 to 1.39; 13 trials, 5815 women).

Local anaesthetic nerve block versus intramuscular analgesia

- One trial, conducted in Denmark (117 women) *(22)*, indicated that the mean time from administering the intervention to the birth was reduced by 37 minutes in the group receiving intramuscular (IM) pethidine versus local anaesthesia (MD 37.00, 95% CI 31.72 to 42.28).

Combined spinal epidural analgesia versus traditional epidural analgesia

- Three trials (> 900 women) that were conducted in the USA, the United Kingdom and France contributed data *(23)*.

- Overall, there was no difference between groups for the number of women requiring augmentation (RR 0.95, 95% CI 0.84 to 1.09).

Combined spinal epidural analgesia versus low-dose epidural analgesia

- Six trials (approximately 500 women) that were conducted in the USA (three), the United Kingdom (two) and Saudi Arabia (one) contributed data *(23)*.

- Overall, there was no significant evidence that the type of epidural (combined spinal versus low-dose) affected the number of women requiring augmentation (more than a third of women in both groups had labour augmentation) (RR 1.00, 95% CI 0.88 to 1.13).

Transcutaneous electrical nerve stimulation (TENS) for pain relief in labour

- Seven trials contributed data, three examining TENS to the back, two TENS to acu-points, one Limoge current to the cranium and one Limoge current to the cranium plus epidural *(24)*.

- There was no significant difference in the number of women requiring augmentation after TENS to the back (RR 0.86, 95% CI 0.59 to 1.25; one trial), TENS to acu-points (RR 0.93, 95% CI 0.78 to 1.11; one trial) or Limoge current to the cranium (RR 0.56, 95% CI 0.29 to 1.07).

- There was also no strong evidence that TENS affected the duration of the first or second stages of labour.

continued...

Recommendation No. 8: Pain relief for preventing delay and reducing the use of augmentation in labour is not recommended. (Weak recommendation, very low quality of evidence)

Relaxation techniques in labour

- A trial conducted in Brazil (36 women) reported that there was a trend towards an increase in the mean length of labour in the relaxation techniques group compared with controls (MD 105.56 min, 95% CI −1.50 to 212.62). A second trial conducted in Italy (34 women) reported no significant difference between groups in the number of women requiring augmentation (RR 1.14, 95% CI 0.82 to 1.59) *(25)*.

Yoga in labour

- Two trials both conducted in Thailand (149 women) reported that the length of labour was reduced in the yoga group (MD −182.19 min, 95% CI −229.68 to −134.70) but that yoga made no difference to the number of women requiring augmentation (approximately half of the women in each group had labour augmentation) (RR 0.76, 95% CI 0.45 to 1.31) *(25)*.

Music in labour

- Although three trials evaluated music and audio-analgesia for pain management during labour, only one of these (60 women), which was conducted in Taiwan, contributed data on duration of first stage of labour *(25)*.

- The length of labour was similar whether or not women had music playing during labour (MD −2.60, 95% CI −11.58 to 6.38).

Acupuncture and acupressure in labour

- Five trials conducted in Northern Europe (four) and Iran (one) contributed data on acupuncture and three trials conducted in Iran, India and Korea contributed data on acupressure *(26)*.

- There was no significant evidence that women who had acupuncture were more or less likely to require augmentation when compared with groups that had placebo (RR 0.62, 95% CI 0.15 to 2.52), standard care (RR 0.88, 95% CI 0.72 to 1.08) or water injection (RR 1.16, 95% CI 0.85 to 1.58).

- There was no significant evidence that acupressure had an effect on the number of women requiring augmentation (RR 0.86, 95% CI 0.69 to 1.06), but acupressure was associated with a reduction in the mean length of labour in two trials (MD −119 min, 95% CI −253.31 to 14.01).

Hypnosis

- Three trials (622 women) conducted in the USA looked at the effect of hypnosis in labour *(27)*. There was a significant difference between groups in the frequency of labour augmentation, with fewer women in the hypnosis group needing this intervention (RR 0.29, 95% CI 0.19 to 0.45).

- In one trial examining hypnosis by a nurse compared with controls there was no significant difference in the number of women requiring labour augmentation (RR 1.06, 95% CI 0.82 to 1.36). Self-hypnosis compared with control appeared to reduce the mean length of labour in one trial with 60 women (MD −165 min, 95% CI −223.53 to −106.87), but self-hypnosis did not appear to affect the need for labour augmentation in another trial (RR 0.98, 95% CI 0.76 to 1.27).

Aromatherapy

- One small trial looked at the effect of aromatherapy on the need for labour augmentation *(28)*. There was no significant difference between groups (RR 1.14, 95% CI 0.90 to 1.45).

Biofeedback

- One trial with a small sample size (55 women) reported no significant difference between groups in the need for labour augmentation with oxytocin (RR 1.19, 95% CI 0.68 to 2.08) when biofeedback was compared with no treatment *(29)*.

Overall quality of evidence

- The quality of the evidence for many outcomes was graded as low or very low (particularly in the trials examining complementary and alternative therapies, many of which had small sample sizes).

> **Recommendation No. 9:** The use of intravenous fluids with the aim of shortening the duration of labour is not recommended. (Strong recommendation, very low quality of evidence)

Remarks

- The GDG did not recommend this intervention on the basis of no clear evidence of benefits over harms. The group noted that the risk of maternal fluid overload, particularly when intravenous oxytocin infusion becomes indicated during the course of labour, may become accentuated.

- The GDG agreed that low-risk women should be encouraged to drink fluids during labour (see Recommendation No. 10 on oral fluid intake in labour).

- The GDG acknowledged that intravenous (IV) fluid may become necessary for other indications and for supportive care in labour even for low-risk women.

- The GDG puts its emphasis on the widespread and unnecessary use of routine administration of IV fluids for all women in labour in many health-care facilities in low-, middle- and high-income settings that increases cost, has considerable impact on the resource use and reduces women's mobility, and therefore made a strong recommendation against this intervention.

Evidence summary: Intravenous fluids for shortening the duration of labour (EB Tables 9a–9h)

- Evidence relating to the use of IV fluids for reducing the duration of labour in low-risk nulliparous women was drawn from a Cochrane systematic review of nine trials (approximately 1700 women) *(30)*. The trials were carried out in the USA (four), Iran (three), Ireland (one) and India (one). The trials examined a range of different comparisons; for most outcomes only one or two trials contributed data.

IV fluids plus oral intake versus oral intake alone: maternal and infant outcomes

- Two trials were included in this comparison.

- The mean duration of labour was reduced by almost half an hour in the women receiving IV fluids (Ringer's lactate) (MD –28.86 min, 95% CI –47.41 to –10.30; two trials, 241 women).

- Compared with oral fluids alone, there was no statistically significant evidence that IV fluids in addition to oral intake affected the rate of caesarean section (RR 0.73, 95% CI 0.49 to 1.08).

- There were no estimable data for maternal fluid overload, and other maternal outcomes were not reported.

- There were no estimable data for low Apgar score at five minutes.

- The event rates for infant admission into NICU were very low and there was no significant difference between comparison groups (RR 0.52, 95% CI 0.05 to 5.59). Other infant outcomes were not reported.

125 ml of IV fluid/hour plus oral intake versus 250 ml IV fluid/hour plus oral intake: maternal and infant outcomes

- The mean duration of labour was reduced by approximately 24 minutes in the group receiving more IV fluid (250 ml) (MD 23.87 min, 95% CI 3.72 to 44.02; three trials, 256 women).

- There were no differences in the number of women undergoing caesarean section (RR 1.00, 95% CI 0.54 to 1.87), although one trial involving 80 women reported fewer assisted vaginal births in the group receiving 125 ml of IV fluid (RR 0.47, 95% CI 0.27 to 0.81).

- There were no estimable data for maternal fluid overload.

- There were no estimable data for low Apgar score at five minutes. The event rates for infant admission into NICU were very low and there was no significant difference between comparison groups (RR 0.56, 95% CI 0.15 to 2.06). Other infant outcomes were not reported.

continued...

> **Recommendation No. 9: The use of intravenous fluids with the aim of shortening the duration of labour is not recommended. (Strong recommendation, very low quality of evidence)**

125 ml IV fluid/hour versus 250 ml IV fluid/hour (restricted oral intake in both arms): maternal and infant outcomes

- The duration of labour appeared shortened in the group receiving more IV fluid (250 ml/hr) (MD 105.61 min, 95% CI 53.19 to 158.02; four trials, 632 women).

- The group receiving more fluid also had a reduced rate of caesarean section (RR 1.56, 95% CI 1.10 to 2.21; four trials, 748 women), although there was no significant difference between groups in the number of assisted vaginal births (RR 0.78, 95% CI 0.44 to 1.40).

- There was one case of fluid overload.

- The event rate was low for low Apgar scores at five minutes, and there was no significant difference between groups. There appeared to be a trend towards more babies with low Apgar scores in the 125 ml/hour group (RR 4.35, 95% CI 0.97 to 19.51; three trials, 689 infants).

- There was no evidence to indicate that the amount of IV fluid affected rates of admission to NICU (RR 0.48, 95% CI 0.07 to 3.17).

Normal saline versus 5% IV dextrose: maternal and infant outcomes

- This comparison included two trials and there were no significant differences between women receiving IV normal saline versus IV 5% dextrose for mean duration of labour (MD –12.00 min, 95% CI –30.09 to 6.09), rate of caesarean section (RR 0.77, 95% CI 0.41 to 1.43) or assisted vaginal birth (RR 0.59, 95% CI 0.21 to 1.63). There were no estimable data for maternal fluid overload.

- In one trial (91 women), maternal hyponatraemia (sodium level < 135 mmol/L) was much more likely in the dextrose group (RR 0.06, 95% CI 0.00 to 0.94).

- There were no significant differences between groups for low Apgar score at five minutes, or admission to NICU. Event rates for both outcomes were low.

- Neonatal hyponatraemia (cord sodium level < 135 mmol/L) was less likely in the normal saline group (RR 0.40, 95% CI 0.17 to 0.93; one trial, 93 infants). There was no difference between groups for neonatal hypoglycaemia.

- Other maternal and neonatal outcomes were not reported.

Overall quality of evidence

- The overall quality of the evidence was graded as very low.

> **Recommendation No. 10: For women at low risk, oral fluid and food intake during labour is recommended. (Weak recommendation, very low quality of evidence)**

Remarks

- Given that restriction of oral fluid and food intake during labour has no beneficial effects on important clinical outcomes including use of labour augmentation, the GDG put its emphasis on respect for the wishes of the woman and therefore made a positive recommendation.

- The GDG noted that no cases of Mendelson's syndrome (inhalation of food and drink from the stomach into the lungs during general anaesthesia – the most important safety concern limiting oral intake during labour) were reported in over 3000 women participating in the trials included in the systematic review.

Evidence summary: Oral fluid and food intake during labour (EB Tables 10a–10h)

- The evidence relating to oral fluid and food intake during labour was extracted from a Cochrane systematic review including five trials (> 3000 women) *(31)*. The trials were conducted in the United Kingdom (three), the Netherlands (one) and Canada (one).

- The trials examined different comparisons: complete restriction of food and drink (other than ice chips) versus freedom to eat and drink at will, water only versus specific food and drink, and water versus carbohydrate drinks (so-called sports drinks). All of the included trials involved women considered to be at low risk of potentially requiring general anaesthesia.

Any restriction of food and drink versus some food and fluid: maternal outcomes

- Three trials (476 women) reported the mean duration of labour associated with restriction of oral intake (other than ice chips). There was no significant difference between the comparison groups (RR –0.29 hrs, 95% CI –1.55 to 0.97) and the findings were inconsistent among the trials.

- All 5 trials (3103 women) reported rates of caesarean section. Again, there were inconsistencies between trials in the size and direction of effect, and overall there was no significant evidence to indicate that restricting food and drink had an effect on the number of women undergoing caesarean section (RR 0.89, 95% CI 0.63 to 1.25).

- There were no significant differences observed between groups in the use of other interventions in labour. The use of epidural analgesia was very similar in both groups (RR 0.98, 95% CI 0.91 to 1.05; 5 trials, 3103 women), as was the rate of labour augmentation (RR 1.02, 95% CI 0.95 to 1.09; 5 trials, 3103 women) and the number of operative vaginal births (RR 0.98, 95% CI 0.88 to 1.10; 5 trials, 3103 women). The use of narcotic pain relief was similar irrespective of restrictions in oral intake (RR 0.94, 95% CI 0.74 to 1.21; 3 trials, 349 women).

- There were no estimable data for the number of women developing Mendelson's syndrome or for any regurgitation during general anaesthesia. Maternal ketonuria was reported in 1 trial (328 women); the rate was very similar in both randomized groups (RR 0.99, 95% CI 0.66 to 1.49). Vomiting during labour was also similar in the 2 groups although there was some inconsistency in results from the trials (RR 0.90, 95% CI 0.62 to 1.31; 3 trials, 2574 women). There was no significant difference between groups for rates of nausea (RR 0.80, 95% CI 0.54 to 1.18; 1 trial, 255 women).

Any restriction of food and drink versus some food and fluid: infant outcomes

- Very few infant outcomes were reported in this review.

- There was no significant difference for low Apgar score at five minutes between groups (RR 1.43, 95% CI 0.77 to 2.68; two trials).

- One trial reported infant admissions to NICU and the frequencies were very similar in both groups (RR 1.03, 95% CI 0.73 to 1.45).

continued...

> **Recommendation No. 10: For women at low risk, oral fluid and food intake during labour is recommended. (Weak recommendation, very low quality of evidence)**

Subgroup analysis

- One trial examined complete restriction of oral food and fluid (other than ice chips) versus freedom to eat and drink and reported similar outcomes for mothers and babies in both groups. There were no significant differences between groups for duration of labour, caesarean section, operative vaginal birth, use of epidural, labour augmentation, or adverse maternal outcomes such as nausea or ketonuria. There were no estimable data for Apgar score at five minutes.

- Similarly, two trials that examined water only versus specific food and drink showed no evidence of differences between the groups for any of the maternal or infant outcomes reported.

- Two trials looked at water versus carbohydrate drinks. Again there was no evidence of significant differences between groups for any of the outcomes reported.

Overall quality

- Overall the quality of the evidence was graded as very low.

> **Recommendation No. 11: Encouraging the adoption of mobility and upright position during labour in women at low risk is recommended. (Strong recommendation, very low quality of evidence)**

Remarks

- Although the evidence does not suggest that mobility and upright position in labour reduce the use of oxytocin augmentation, the GDG placed its emphasis on the clinical benefits in term of reducing caesarean section.

- GDG noted that in many settings, traditional practices of enforcing bed rest for all women in labour are common, rather than allowing women's choices to be informed by their knowledge of the benefits of mobility and upright position. The GDG put its emphasis on providing women with the choice of an intervention that is beneficial, cheap and easy to implement, and therefore made a strong recommendation for this intervention.

- This recommendation should inform and support women's choices on what position to adopt during the first stage of labour.

- The GDG was informed of a large, ongoing trial in the United Kingdom, which is examining maternal position in women with epidural analgesia during labour.

> **Evidence summary: Maternal position and mobility during the first stage of labour for improving outcomes (EB Tables 11a–11d)**

- Evidence relating to mobility and upright position compared with bed care for women in labour was extracted from a Cochrane systematic review of 25 trials (> 5000 women) *(32)*. The review included both randomized and quasi-randomized controlled trials. Most of the women recruited into the trials were at full term with no pregnancy complications. About half of the included trials recruited only nulliparous women and a subgroup analysis by parity was performed. The trials examined two different comparisons: upright and ambulant care versus bed care for women with (seven trials) and without (18 trials) epidural analgesia at the point of randomization.

- Trials were conducted in a range of high-, middle- and low-resource countries, including five in the USA, seven in the United Kingdom, two in France, and one trial each in Australia, Brazil, China, China, Hong Kong Special Administrative Region, Finland, Japan, India, Iran, Sweden, Thailand, and Tunisia.

- A very broad range of interventions was considered in this review; upright and ambulant positions ranged from women sitting, kneeling, squatting and walking, through to taking up other positions either on or off the bed. Compliance was poor in some trials with women choosing to take up whatever position they were comfortable with.

Upright and ambulant positions for women without epidural: maternal outcomes

- The duration of the first stage of labour was on average 1.36 hours shorter in the upright and ambulant group (95% CI −2.22 to −0.51; 15 trials, 2503 women) compared to supine and recumbent position. There was inconsistency in the size and direction of effect and high statistical heterogeneity for this outcome. The overall result favoured the upright group in both nulliparous and multiparous women; however, fewer trials examined this outcome for multiparous women and the difference for this subgroup was not significant (nulliparous: MD −1.21 hrs, 95% CI −2.35 to −0.07; 12 trials, 1486 women; multiparous: MD −0.56 hrs, 95% CI −1.19 to 0.06; four trials, 662 women).

- There were no significant differences overall or in subgroups for the duration of the second stage of labour, but there was inconsistency in the size and direction of effect in different trials (overall MD −2.29 min, 95% CI −6.49 to 1.91; nine trials, 2077 women).

- Women in the upright and ambulant groups were less likely to undergo caesarean section (RR 0.71, 95% CI 0.54 to 0.94; 14 trials, 2682 women). But there were no significant differences between groups for spontaneous vaginal birth (overall RR 1.05, 95% CI 0.99 to 1.11) or operative vaginal birth (overall RR 0.91, 95% CI 0.73 to 1.14).

continued...

> **Recommendation No. 11:** Encouraging the adoption of mobility and upright position during labour in women at low risk is recommended. (Strong recommendation, very low quality of evidence)

Upright and ambulant positions for women without epidural: maternal outcomes (continued)

- There was a modest reduction in the number of women using epidural analgesia among women in the upright and ambulant groups (RR 0.81, 95% CI 0.66 to 0.99; nine trials, 2107 women).

- No significant difference was observed between groups in the frequency of labour augmentation (RR 0.89, 95% CI 0.76 to 1.05; eight trials, 1826 women).

- Only two trials (240 women) reported on PPH; there were few events and no significant differences between groups (RR 0.71, 95% CI 0.14 to 3.55).

- Other critical maternal outcomes were not reported.

Upright and ambulant positions for women without epidural: infant outcomes

- Few critical and important infant outcomes were reported. For most outcomes event rates were low and estimates imprecise. There were no significant differences between women that were upright and ambulant versus those lying in bed during labour for perinatal mortality (RR 0.50, 95% CI 0.05 to 5.37); fetal distress leading to immediate delivery (RR 0.69, 95% CI 0.35 to 1.33); Apgar score < 7 at five minutes (RR 3.27, 95% CI 0.34 to 31.05); need for intubation at birth (RR 0.77, 95% CI 0.19 to 3.10); or admission to NICU (RR 0.58, 95% CI 0.25 to 1.36).

- Other critical or important infant outcomes were not reported.

Upright and ambulant positions for women with epidural: maternal outcomes

- For women with epidural analgesia, there was no significant difference between groups for mode of delivery either overall or in parity subgroups: caesarean section (overall RR 1.05, 95% CI 0.83 to 1.32); spontaneous vaginal birth (overall RR 0.96, 95% CI 0.89 to 1.05); operative vaginal birth (overall RR 1.06, 95% CI 0.9 to 1.25).

- The duration of the second stage of labour was reported in two trials and there was no evidence of any difference between groups (MD 2.35 min, 95% CI −15.22 to 19.91).

- The number of women requiring labour augmentation was high in both groups (more than half) and maternal position or mobility did not have a significant effect on this outcome (RR 0.98, 95% CI 0.90 to 1.07).

- Other critical maternal outcomes were not reported.

Upright and ambulant positions for women with epidural: infant outcomes

- Only one infant outcome was reported. Four trials reported the number of babies with low Apgar scores at five minutes, but only two trials had estimable data and there was no significant difference between groups (RR 1.04, 95% CI 0.21 to 5.05); event rates were very low in the other two trials.

Overall quality of evidence:

- For both comparisons, the quality of the evidence was graded as low or very low for most outcomes, and due to the low event rates for most of the neonatal outcomes many of the effect estimates relating to the condition of the newborn were imprecise.

Recommendation No. 12: Continuous companionship during labour is recommended for improving labour outcomes. (Strong recommendation, moderate quality of evidence)

Remarks

- The GDG acknowledged that continuous psychosocial support may not necessarily reduce the need for labour augmentation but made the recommendation on the basis of other substantial benefits for women and their babies.

- The GDG noted that countries and policy-makers are often reluctant to implement this intervention in practice in spite of the supporting evidence, which has been available for many years. The group agreed that extra efforts are needed to encourage potential implementers at various levels of health care delivery.

- The GDG discussed the issues of privacy, cultural inclinations and resource use often raised as concerns to implementing this intervention and agreed that simple measures to allow female relatives to accompany women during labour could be used as cost-effective and culturally sensitive ways to address these concerns.

- The evidence supports the use of any type of culturally appropriate companion, including husband and lay professionals, such as doulas.

Evidence summary: Continuous companionship during labour for improving labour outcomes (EB Tables 12a–12b)

- Evidence was extracted from a Cochrane systematic review of 22 trials (> 15 000 women) *(33)*. The trials were conducted in low-, middle- and high-income countries across the world (USA, Canada, Belgium, France, Greece, Finland, Sweden, South Africa, Botswana, Nigeria, Australia, Brazil, Thailand, Mexico, Guatemala, Chile and Iran). Hospital routines and facilities varied considerably in different settings; for example, epidural analgesia was not routinely available in seven of the trials.

- Continuous support was defined slightly differently in different trials but mainly women were accompanied at least during the active stages of labour. The companions in different trials varied: sometimes labour companions (or doulas) provided support while in other trials a female relative or husband was present throughout labour.

Continuous support versus usual care: maternal outcomes

- The mean length of labour was reduced for women supported in labour by approximately 35 minutes (MD –0.58 hrs, 95% CI –0.85 to –0.31; 12 trials, 5366 women).

- The rate of operative deliveries was reduced if they were supported during labour. The rate of caesarean section was reduced by more than 20% (RR 0.78, 95% CI 0.67 to 0.91; 22 trials, 15 175 women) and there was a modest reduction in the number of women undergoing instrumental vaginal birth (RR 0.90, 95% CI 0.85 to 0.96, 19 trials, 14 118 women), so that the overall number of women with spontaneous vaginal births was increased (RR 1.08, 95% CI 1.04 to 1.12; 19 trials, 14 119 women).

- There was a slight reduction in other interventions in labour in the supported group. The use of regional analgesia was reduced by approximately 7% (RR 0.93, 95% CI 0.88 to 0.99; nine trials, 11 444 women) and the number of women requiring other analgesia was also reduced (RR 0.90, 95% CI 0.84 to 0.96; 14 trials, 12 283 women).

- There was no significant difference between groups in the requirement of synthetic oxytocin during labour. Overall, more than a third of women in both groups received oxytocin (RR 0.97, 95% CI 0.91 to 1.04; 15 trials, 12 620 women), although there was considerable variation between trials.

- Only two trials reported on postpartum depression and results suggested that continuous support was associated with lower rates of depression. The two trials were carried out in very different settings and outcomes were measured in different ways, and while the direction of the effect was the same, the size of the effect was very different so results were not pooled.

continued...

> **Recommendation No. 12: Continuous companionship during labour is recommended for improving labour outcomes. (Strong recommendation, moderate quality of evidence)**
>
> *Continuous support versus usual care: maternal outcomes (continued)*
>
> - More than half of the women in both groups had perineal trauma and there was no significant difference between groups (RR 0.97, 95% CI 0.92 to 1.01).
>
> - Women were much less likely to report negative feelings about their childbirth experience if they received continuous support (RR 0.69, 95% CI 0.59 to 0.79; 11 trials, 11 133 women).
>
> *Continuous support versus usual care: infant outcomes*
>
> - Infants whose mothers had been supported were less likely to have an Apgar score < 7 at five minutes (RR 0.69, 95% CI 0.50 to 0.95; 13 trials, 12 515 infants).
>
> - There were no clear differences in the number of babies admitted for special care or having prolonged hospital stays (RR 0.97, 95% CI 0.76 to 1.25, and RR 0.83, 95% CI 0.42 to 1.65 respectively).
>
> - Continuous support did not seem to affect the number of babies being breastfed at 1–2 months postpartum, although this outcome was only reported in three trials (RR 1.01, 95% CI 0.94 to 1.09).
>
> *Overall quality of evidence*
>
> - The overall quality of the evidence was graded as moderate.

Recommendation No. 13: Administration of enema for reducing the use of labour augmentation is not recommended. (Strong recommendation, very low quality of evidence)

Remarks

- The GDG noted that the routine use of enema has neither been shown to reduce the duration of labour nor confer any other clinical benefits. It is considered invasive and associated with discomfort for women.

- The GDG put its emphasis on the feasibility of implementing this recommendation, the reduction in health resource use and acceptability by caregivers and women and therefore made a strong recommendation against this intervention.

Evidence summary: Routine enema for improving labour outcomes (EB Tables 13a–13b)

- Evidence was drawn from a Cochrane systematic review of four trials (almost 2000 women) *(34)*, although for most of the outcomes reported, data were available from only one or two trials. The trials were conducted in the USA, Thailand, Colombia and the United Kingdom.

- Few critical and important maternal and infant outcomes were reported and overall, there were no significant differences between groups.

Enema versus no enema: maternal outcomes

- Two trials (1179 women) reported on the total duration of labour; no statistically significant difference was observed in the duration of labour (MD 28.04 min, 95% CI –131.01 to 187.10) but there was a high level of heterogeneity between the findings of the two trials.

- There was also no observed difference between groups regarding the duration of the second stage of labour (MD 5.2 min, 95% CI –2.56 to 12.96).

- No significant differences were observed in the rates of second or third degree perineal trauma (RR 0.68, 95% CI 0.39 to 1.21). Intrapartum infection was marginally increased among women who received routine exnema (RR 4.62, 95% CI 1.03 to 20.68) but women requiring systemic antibiotics following the birth were similar between the two comparison groups (RR 1.16, 95% CI 0.73 to 1.84; one trial, 428 women).

- One trial (1027 women) reported women's level of satisfaction with childbirth (measured on a Likert scale but reported as a continuous outcome): the mean scores were identical in the two groups (MD 0.00, 95% CI –0.10 to 0.10).

Enema versus no enema: infant outcomes

- The review reported very little information on infant outcomes. There was no significant difference in the rate of infants with low Apgar scores at five minutes (RR 1.31, 95% CI 0.57 to 3.06). Rates of neonatal infection (variously defined) were similar between the groups (RR 0.61, 95% CI 0.24 to 1.52).

Overall quality of evidence

- The overall quality of evidence was graded as very low.

3.3.3 Treatment of delay in the first stage of labour with augmentation

> **Recommendation No. 14:** The use of oxytocin alone for treatment of delay in labour is recommended.
> *(Weak recommendation, very low quality of evidence)*

Remarks

- The GDG noted that there is insufficient evidence to demonstrate the benefits of oxytocin augmentation for delayed labour, in spite of its widespread use in clinical practice. However, it was agreed that the ability of oxytocin to stimulate uterine contractions both before and during labour is undisputed and judicious oxytocin use in case of insufficient contractions can prevent unduly prolonged labour.

- The recommendation leaned on the evidence of some benefits of oxytocin when used as a single intervention for labour induction, compared with expectant management, and by inference the potential for benefit where the primary cause of delay in labour progress is insufficient uterine contractions.

Evidence summary: Oxytocin (alone) for treatment of slow progress in the first stage of labour (EB Tables 14a–14b)

- Evidence on the use of oxytocin versus placebo or no treatment for delayed progress in labour was drawn from a Cochrane systematic review of three trials (138 women) conducted in Thailand, Argentina and the USA *(35)*. Women recruited into the trials were described as being at low risk, with term pregnancies and in the first stage of spontaneous labour. Almost all of the women included in the trials were nulliparous.

IV oxytocin versus no treatment: maternal outcomes

- The review reported none of the critical outcomes, and provided data for very few important outcomes.

- There were no significant differences between women randomized to receive oxytocin versus women in the control group for caesarean section (RR 0.84, 95% CI 0.36 to 1.96) or instrumental vaginal birth (RR 1.04, 95% CI 0.45 to 2.41).

IV oxytocin versus no treatment: infant outcomes

- For low Apgar score at five minutes, there were no events in either group (one trial, 87 women).

Overall quality of evidence

- Evidence available regarding oxytocin compared to no treatment is insufficient to support any conclusions about its benefits or harms. The overall quality of the evidence was graded as very low.

- Evidence on the use of oxytocin along with other interventions (e.g. amniotomy) or as part of a package of care for the active management of labour is presented separately.

> **Recommendation No. 15: Augmentation with intravenous oxytocin prior to confirmation of delay in labour is not recommended. (Weak recommendation, very low quality of evidence)**

Remarks

- The GDG noted that the clinical benefits of immediate, compared to delayed, commencement of oxytocin following a suspicion of slow labour progress do not clearly outweigh its potential harms.

- The GDG members placed emphasis on the need to confirm a delay in the progress of labour by allowing an interval of watchful expectancy before initiating oxytocin augmentation. The GDG members agreed such a course of action could reduce the frequency of premature diagnosis of labour dystocia and unnecessary oxytocin augmentation. Furthermore, early intervention on the basis of suspected labour dystocia may be associated with more uterine hyperstimulation and poorer maternal and neonatal morbidity in settings where interventions to manage the condition are not available.

Evidence summary: Early versus delayed use of oxytocin for treatment of slow progress in the first stage of labour (EB Tables 15a–15b)

- Evidence on early use of oxytocin versus delayed use during the first stage of labour was drawn from a Cochrane systematic review of five trials (1200 low-risk women) *(35)*. Women recruited into the trials were described as being at low risk, with term pregnancies and in the first stage of spontaneous labour. Almost all of the women included in the trials were nulliparous. Three trials were conducted in the United Kingdom and one each in Sweden and Finland.

- Women recruited into "early" oxytocin groups in the trials received oxytocin immediately or within 20 minutes following the diagnosis of delay in labour progress. Those in the "delayed" oxytocin group received more conservative management with oxytocin augmentation withheld for a variable time period of between three and eight hours following diagnosis of delay in labour progress.

- Diagnosis of slow progress in the first stage of labour was heterogeneous among trials.

Early versus delayed use of oxytocin: maternal outcomes

- Women receiving early oxytocin had, on average, a shorter interval between randomization and birth (MD 2.2 hrs shorter, 95% CI –3.29 to –1.1; three trials, 1083 women). There was considerable variation in the size of the effect between the three trials reporting this outcome, but the direction of effect was consistent. Two trials indicated no significant difference between the comparison groups in the number of women undelivered 12 hours after randomization (RR 0.32, 95% CI 0.07 to 1.43; two trials, 1042 women).

- Women in the early oxytocin group were more likely to have uterine hyperstimulation with fetal heart rate changes (RR 2.51, 95% CI 1.04 to 6.05; two trials, 472 women). However, one small trial (60 women) failed to show an effect between groups for uterine hyperstimulation without fetal heart rate changes (RR 6.66, 95% CI 0.39 to 112.6).

- There was no significant difference between groups for incidence of PPH (RR 0.83, 95% CI 0.59 to 1.15; three trials, 1099 women).

- The mode of delivery was similar between the groups. A similar proportion of women in the early and delayed oxytocin groups had caesarean section for any indication (RR 0.88, 95% CI 0.66 and 1.19; five trials, 1200 women), and caesarean section for fetal distress (RR 1.08, 95% CI 0.59 to 2.0; three trials, 909 women). There were no differences observed in the number of women having instrumental vaginal birth (RR 1.17, 95% CI 0.72 to 1.88; five trials, 1200 women) or using epidural analgesia (RR 0.9, 95% CI 0.76 to 1.06; three trials, 1083 women).

- Two trials that collected information on women's views of their experiences in childbirth indicated no differences in maternal satisfaction between the groups.

continued...

> **Recommendation No. 15: Augmentation with intravenous oxytocin prior to confirmation of delay in labour is not recommended. (Weak recommendation, very low quality of evidence)**
>
> *Early versus delayed use of oxytocin: infant outcomes*
>
> - There were no significant differences between groups for any of the neonatal outcomes reported. Serious neonatal morbidity or perinatal death was reported in two trials, and overall there were only two events (one in each group). There were similarities between groups regarding low Apgar scores at five minutes (RR 1.02, 95% CI 0.46 to 2.28), and admission to NICU (RR 0.95, 95% CI 0.60 to 1.50).
>
> *Overall quality of evidence*
>
> - The overall quality of the evidence for early versus delayed use of oxytocin was graded as very low.
>
> - Evidence on the use of oxytocin along with other interventions (e.g. amniotomy) or as part of a package of care for the active management of labour is presented separately.

> **Recommendation No. 16: High starting and increment dosage regimen of oxytocin is not recommended for labour augmentation. (Weak recommendation, very low quality of evidence)**
>
> **Remarks**
>
> - The GDG considered the evidence in favour of high starting and increment dosage regimen of oxytocin (in terms of labour duration and overall caesarean section rate) to be uncertain and chose not to recommend the intervention. The group emphasised the need for caution in initiating and increasing oxytocin at high dosage levels, given the paucity of evidence on critical neonatal outcomes and the danger associated with injudicious use of oxytocin in clinical practice.
>
> **Evidence summary: High versus low oxytocin dosage regimen for labour augmentation (EB Tables 16a–16b)**
>
> - Evidence on the use of high- versus low-dose oxytocin regimens was drawn from one Cochrane systematic review including four trials (644 women) *(36)*.
> - Two of the trials recruited nulliparous women only. High-dose regimens were defined as those with starting doses and increments of ≥ four milliunit (mU) per minute of oxytocin, and low-dose regimens as those with a starting dose and increments of < four mU per minute. The division into "high" and "low" doses was based on an arbitrary decision.
> - Two of the trials were conducted in the United Kingdom and one trial each was conducted in the USA and Iran.
>
> *High- versus low-dose oxytocin: maternal outcomes*
>
> - In one trial (92 women) there was no significant difference between the high- and low-dose groups for the mean interval from onset of the first stage of labour to delivery (MD –26 min, 95% CI –128.06 to 76.06) while in another trial (40 women), the mean interval from the start of oxytocin administration to delivery was reduced by 3.5 hours in the higher-dose group (95% CI –6.38 to –0.62).
> - There was no significant difference between groups in the incidence of PPH (RR 0.95, 95% CI 0.61 to 1.48).
> - For caesarean section, there was a significant difference between groups, with the high-dose group being less likely to undergo caesarean section (RR 0.62, 95% CI 0.44 to 0.86; four trials, 644 women). However, there was inconsistency between trials in the size of the effect, and more than half of the weight in this analysis was from a trial at high risk of bias; when this trial was excluded from the analysis, the observed difference between groups was not statistically significant, and the effect size was considerably reduced (RR 0.89, 95% CI 0.57 to 1.38). The above results were reflected in the rate of spontaneous vaginal birth, which favoured the high-dose group (RR 1.35, 95% CI 1.13 to 1.62), but again this was largely due to the data from a single trial at high risk of bias. There was no significant difference in the rate of instrumental vaginal births (RR 0.83, 95% CI 0.61 to 1.13).
> - No significant difference was observed between groups for uterine hyperstimulation, although there was a trend towards an increased risk among women receiving a high dose of oxytocin for labour augmentation (RR 1.63, 95% CI 0.97 to 2.72; four trials, 644 women). Use of epidural analgesia was very similar in the two groups (RR 0.98, 95% CI 0.86 to 1.12).
> - There was no significant difference between groups for chorioamnionitis (RR 0.7, 95% CI 0.44 to 1.12).
>
> *High- versus low-dose oxytocin: infant outcomes*
>
> - Few data on neonatal outcomes were reported. There were no estimable data to show an effect in neonatal mortality or Apgar score < 7 at five minutes. No significant differences were observed for mean umbilical cord artery pH (MD 0, 95% CI –0.03 to 0.03) or admission to NICU (RR 0.5, 95% CI 0.22 to 1.15).
>
> *Overall quality of evidence*
>
> - The overall quality of the evidence was rated as very low.
> - The use of oxytocin versus no active treatment and its use with other interventions is presented separately.

Recommendation No. 17: The use of oral misoprostol for labour augmentation is not recommended. (Strong recommendation, very low quality of evidence)
Remarks

- The GDG noted that there is no clear evidence that the potential benefits of oral misoprostol, compared to intravenous oxytocin, for labour augmentation outweigh its potential harms.

- The GDG concluded that oral misoprostol is unlikely to be a safe substitute to oxytocin for labour augmentation where skilled attendants are available. The group also noted that settings where skilled birth attendants are not available (and where misoprostol could have been useful in this regard) are also likely to lack the resources to manage complications that could arise in women undergoing augmentation.

- The GDG considers the dosage regimens used in the primary studies as not evidence based with potential for serious harms, given the high rate of uterine hyperstimulation with fetal heart rate changes. The group put its emphasis on the implications of such adverse effects for maternal and infant outcomes, particularly in low-resource settings, and therefore strengthened the recommendation.

- Further pharmacological effects of orally ingested misoprostol, if found detrimental to the health of the mother or her baby during the course of labour, cannot be prevented by termination of the therapy as is possible with oxytocin infusion.

Evidence summary: Oral misoprostol for augmenting labour (EB Table 17a–17d)

- Evidence was drawn from a Cochrane systematic review that included two trials, each examining a different comparison *(37)*. Women in both trials were all in spontaneous labour requiring augmentation. The trials were conducted in Taiwan and the USA.

- The trial in Taiwan, China (231 women) compared titrated oral misoprostol with IV oxytocin for labour augmentation. Women in the misoprostol group were randomized to receive an initial dose of 20 micrograms (mcg) of misoprostol (in 20 ml of water) repeated every hour up to four hours, after which the dose was increased to 40 mcg per hour up to a maximum cumulative dose of 1600 mcg. All but three of the women randomized received the intended treatment.

- In the trial in the USA, women were randomized to receive either oral misoprostol or usual care (IV oxytocin). In this trial, lower doses of misoprostol were achieved by cutting up 100 mcg tablets. Women were initially given 75 mcg of oral misoprostol, which was repeated after four hours provided no adverse effects were observed. There was considerable deviation from protocol in this trial although analysis was by intention to treat: in the misoprostol group 136/176 (77.3%) received the trial drug, while in the oxytocin group 143/174 (82.2%) women received the control drug as intended.

- Findings for the two trials were not pooled in view of the different misoprostol regimens.

Titrated oral misoprostol versus oxytocin: maternal outcomes

- For the misoprostol group on the 20 mcg per hour regimen, overall there was no evidence of differences between groups for most critical and important maternal outcomes.

- Mode of delivery was similar in the misoprostol and oxytocin groups; most of the women in both groups gave birth vaginally within 24 hours of the commencement of augmentation (RR 1.02, 95% CI 0.93 to 1.11). Similar numbers of women (approximately 80% in both groups) had given birth vaginally within 12 hours of augmentation (RR 0.91, 95% CI 0.80 to 1.03). There was no significant difference between groups in terms of the number of women undergoing caesarean section (RR 0.88, 95% CI 0.42 to 1.85). Rates of "failure to progress" were similar in the two groups (RR 0.80, 95% CI 0.36 to 1.77).

continued...

> **Recommendation No. 17: The use of oral misoprostol for labour augmentation is not recommended. (Strong recommendation, very low quality of evidence)**
>
> *Titrated oral misoprostol versus oxytocin: maternal outcomes (continued)*
>
> - Few women (two in each group) had uterine hyperstimulation with fetal heart rate changes (RR 0.96, 95% CI 0.14 to 6.68). No women were identified with hypertonus, but more women in the oxytocin group were reported to have tachysystole: 7/118 in the misoprostol group versus 17/113 in the oxytocin group (RR 0.39, 95% CI 0.17 to 0.91).
>
> - Maternal side-effects (including pyrexia, shivering, nausea and vomiting) were reported, but there were very few events in either group.
>
> - For the 75-mcg dosage regimen, there was no evidence of differences between groups for most maternal outcomes.
>
> - There were no significant differences between women in the misoprostol and oxytocin groups for rate of caesarean section for fetal distress (RR 1.58, 95% CI 0.53 to 4.74), caesarean section for prolonged labour (RR 0.84, 95% CI 0.39 to 1.82), or caesarean section for any indication (RR 1.04, 95% CI 0.57 to 1.92). Few women had forceps delivery (RR 1.98, 95% CI 0.37 to 10.66) and the overall rate of spontaneous vaginal birth was very similar in both groups (RR 0.98, 95% CI 0.91 to 1.06).
>
> - More than a quarter of women in both groups were reported to have uterine hyperstimulation with fetal heart rate changes and, although the rate was higher in the misoprostol group, the difference between the groups was not statistically significant (RR 1.26, 95% CI 0.88 to 1.80). Uterine hyperstimulation over a 10-minute period (without fetal heart rate changes) was reported for more than 60% of women in both groups; more women in the misoprostol group (approximately 75% versus 64%) were reported to have hyperstimulation of labour (RR 1.17, 95% CI 1.02 to 1.35). The number of women with tachysystole over a 20-minute observation period was reported to be similar in both groups (RR 1.21, 95% CI 0.84 to 1.72).
>
> - Most of the women in both groups had epidural analgesia (RR 0.92, 95% CI 0.84 to 1.01). Maternal blood transfusion for hypovolemia was reported, and no difference between groups was identified (RR 2.97, 95% CI 0.61 to 14.49). Rates of chorioamnionitis were similar for the women in both groups (RR 0.87, 95% CI 0.55 to 1.37).
>
> *Titrated oral misoprostol versus oxytocin: infant outcomes*
>
> - For the 20-mcg dosage regimen, few important infant outcomes were reported.
>
> - There were no babies with Apgar scores < 7 at five minutes in either group. There were few admissions to NICU, and no significant difference between groups (RR 2.39, 95% CI 0.47 to 12.09).
>
> - For the 75-mcg dosage regimen, Apgar score of < 4 at five minutes was reported: there were no events in either group. Only one baby was admitted to NICU. There was no significant difference between groups for umbilical cord artery pH of < 7.1 (RR 0.74, 95% CI 0.17 to 3.26). Other critical and important neonatal outcomes were not reported.
>
> *Overall quality of evidence*
>
> - Overall quality of evidence for reported outcomes was graded as very low, mainly due to imprecision resulting from the small sample sizes and low event rates for many outcomes.

Recommendation No. 18: The use of amniotomy alone for treatment of delay in labour is not recommended. (Weak recommendation, very low quality of evidence)

Remarks

- The GDG noted that the lack of sufficient evidence to conclude on the benefits or harms of amniotomy alone for the treatment of delay in labour in spite of its common use in clinical practice.

- While acknowledging the lack of evidence regarding the benefits of amniotomy as a treatment intervention for confirmed delay in labour progress, the GDG noted that the decision to rupture the membranes could be made on the basis of other considerations, such as the need for fetal monitoring.

- This recommendation may be stronger for HIV-positive women and those with unknown HIV status in HIV prevalent settings, where delayed rupture of membranes is beneficial in terms of reducing the risk of perinatal HIV transmission.

Evidence summary: The use of routine amniotomy alone for treatment of delay in the first stage of labour (EB Tables 18a–18b)

- Evidence related to the use of amniotomy alone to treat delay in the first stage of spontaneous labour was drawn from one Cochrane systematic review that included one trial (40 women) conducted in the United Kingdom comparing amniotomy versus intention to preserve amniotic membranes *(19)*.

- Women were recruited when labour was diagnosed not to be progressing satisfactorily using a partogram.

- Most of the critical and important outcomes were not reported.

Routine amniotomy versus intention to preserve amniotic membranes (no routine amniotomy): maternal outcomes

- There were no maternal deaths in either group.

- No indicators of serious maternal morbidity were reported.

- There were no observed differences in the rates of caesarean section for any indication (RR 0.95, 95% CI 0.15 to 6.08), caesarean section for fetal distress (RR 2.86, 95% CI 0.12 to 66.11) or caesarean section for prolonged labour (RR 0.47, 95% CI 0.05 to 4.82).

Routine amniotomy versus intention to preserve amniotic membranes (no routine amniotomy): infant outcomes

- Reported neonatal outcomes were limited to Apgar score < 7 at five minutes and admission to NICU. Both outcomes were similar between the comparison groups.

Overall quality of evidence

- Overall, the quality of the available evidence was graded as very low. The available data are insufficient to draw conclusions on the benefits or harms of routine amniotomy for treatment of dysfunctional labour.

Recommendation No. 19: The use of amniotomy and oxytocin for treatment of confirmed delay in labour is recommended. (Weak recommendation, very low quality of evidence)

Remarks

- The GDG agreed that, despite the lack of research evidence, if a delay in labour progress is associated with lack of regular uterine contractions, the stimulation of uterine contractions with oxytocin and amniotomy is a reasonable clinical choice. The group acknowledged the lack of evidence on how the sequence of amniotomy and oxytocin infusion affects outcomes and considers this a research priority.
- There is a need to exercise caution among women with HIV.

Evidence summary: Amniotomy and oxytocin for treatment of delay in the first stage of labour (EB Tables 19a–19b)

- Evidence on the use of amniotomy and oxytocin compared with routine care for the treatment of delay was drawn from one Cochrane systematic review including three RCTs (280 women) *(17)*. Two of the trials were conducted in the United Kingdom and one was conducted in Israel.
- Women with established delay in the first stage of labour were allocated to amniotomy and oxytocin versus usual care. Usual care varied across different settings.

Amniotomy and oxytocin for the treatment of delay: maternal outcomes

- The review did not report on maternal mortality.
- There was a significant reduction in the total duration of labour for women in the intervention group in one trial (MD –3.10 hrs, 95% CI –4.63 to –1.57; 141 women). However, two trials failed to demonstrate a difference in the length of the first stage of labour (MD –1.58 hrs, 95% CI –4.27 to 1.10; 240 women).
- There was no significant difference between groups in the frequency of PPH (blood loss > 500 ml) (RR 6.90, 95% CI 0.36 to 131.23; one trial, 141 women).
- There was no significant difference between groups for rates of caesarean section for any indication (RR 1.47, 95% CI 0.73 to 2.96; three trials, 280 women) or spontaneous vaginal birth (RR 0.96, 95% CI 0.85 to 1.08; three trials, 282 women).
- There were no reported data on hyperstimulation of labour or maternal blood transfusion.
- One trial reported comparable maternal satisfaction with labour experience in both groups (RR 1.02, 95% CI 0.75 to 1.39).
- One trial reported rates of maternal fever or infection: event rates were low and there was no difference between groups (RR 1.63, 95% CI 0.41 to 6.47).

Amniotomy and oxytocin for the treatment of delay: infant outcomes

- For neonatal outcomes, there were no data on serious neonatal morbidity, abnormal arterial cord pH (acidosis), jaundice or hyperbilirubinaemia.
- The trials were too small to show a difference between groups for admission to NICU (RR 0.08, 95% CI 0.00 to 1.30; one trial, 99 women) or Apgar score < 7 at five minutes (RR 2.73, 95% CI 0.12 to 63.19; one trial, 40 women); event rates for both outcomes were very low and effect estimates were therefore imprecise.

Overall quality of evidence

- Overall, the quality of the evidence was graded as low or very low, and the combined sample size of the three trials contributing data was less than 300. There was a paucity of evidence for neonatal outcomes.
- Evidence relating to the use of amniotomy alone, oxytocin alone and both amniotomy and oxytocin as part of a package of care for active management of labour is presented separately.

3.3.4 Care during labour augmentation

> **Recommendation No. 20:** The use of internal tocodynamometry, compared with external tocodynamometry, with the aim of improving outcomes for augmented labour is not recommended. (Weak recommendation, very low quality of evidence)

Remarks

- The GDG noted that there is no evidence to suggest that the potential benefits of internal, compared with external, tocodynamometry in women undergoing labour augmentation clearly outweighs its potential harms. The group did not recommend one method over the other but noted that internal tocodynamometry is resource-intensive and currently not widely practiced in many settings.

- The GDG stressed the importance of ensuring that every woman undergoing labour augmentation should receive regular and frequent monitoring of uterine contraction pattern and fetal heart rate, within the limits of available resources.

Evidence summary: Internal versus external tocodynamometry in augmented labour (EB Tables 20a–20b)

- Findings were extracted from a Cochrane systematic review that included two trials (750 women) *(38)*. The trials were conducted in Singapore and the Netherlands. The trial in the Netherlands also recruited women who had undergone labour induction, but the data on women who had had their labour augmented were provided separately.

- Comparing internal versus external tocodynamometry, few outcomes showed statistically significant differences between groups for maternal and infant outcomes.

Internal versus external tocodynamometry in augmented labour: maternal outcomes

- The mean time to vaginal birth was very similar for women monitored by internal or external tocodynamometry (MD −3.47 min, 95% CI −42.84 to 35.90; one trial, 500 women).

- There were no estimable data for serious maternal morbidity (including uterine rupture) or maternal death.

- There were no ignificant differences between groups for caesarean section (RR 1.25, 95% CI 0.91 to 1.71; two trials, 750 women) or instrumental vaginal birth (RR 1.25, 95% CI 0.91 to 1.73; two trials, 750 women). For all operative deliveries (caesarean section and instrumental vaginal births combined), the difference between groups was statistically significant with a marginally increased risk in the internal tocodynamometry group (RR 1.25, 95% CI 1.02 to 1.53; two trials, 750 women).

- Uterine hyperstimulation was reported in only one trial (250 women) and the rate was very similar in both groups (RR 1.04, 95% CI 0.63 to 1.72).

- There was no significant difference between groups for maternal intrauterine infection requiring antibiotic therapy (RR 0.55, 95% CI 0.26 to 1.16; one trial, 500 women).

Internal versus external tocodynamometry in augmented labour: infant outcomes

- There were no estimable data for several infant outcomes including perinatal mortality and adverse events such as placental or fetal blood vessel damage. There were very few babies with low Apgar scores at five minutes in either group (overall 15/749) and no statistically significant difference between groups (RR 1.12, 95% CI 0.41 to 3.06).

- Umbilical cord artery pH of < 7.05 and < 7.15 were reported in one trial: there was no significant difference between groups at either cut-off (RR 1.13, 95% CI 0.39 to 3.30, and RR 1.38, 95% CI 0.88 to 2.15, respectively).

- There was no significant difference between women undergoing internal versus external tocodynamometry for admission of infants to NICU (RR 1.00, 95% CI 0.06 to 15.81) or for prolonged NICU stay (> 48 hrs) (RR 0.83, 95% CI 0.51 to 1.35).

Overall quality of evidence

- The overall quality of the evidence was graded as very low.

4. Research implications

The Guideline Development Group (GDG) identified important gaps in existing knowledge that need to be addressed through primary research. It was observed that despite the increasing practice of augmentation of labour worldwide, the paucity of strong evidence was striking. The quality of evidence was rated as low or very low for most of the recommendations. From the GRADE methodology standpoint, evidence rated as low or very low quality implies that further research is likely to have an impact on the corresponding recommendations. Conversely, further research is not a priority for those recommendations based on evidence of moderate or high quality. The knowledge gaps identified based on this concept were prioritized by considering whether such research would be original, innovative, feasible, and likely to promote equity and to contribute to improvement in intrapartum care.

The GDG acknowledged that in spite of the lack of clear benefits for certain interventions that are deeply embedded in clinical practice (e.g. oxytocin alone for augmentation), initiation of rigorous primary studies is likely to face significant ethical and recruitment challenges.

4.1 Key research priorities

- What are the comparative effects of oxytocin alone, amniotomy alone and concurrent oxytocin and amniotomy in women with confirmed delay in the first stage of labour?
    - » How does the sequence of oxytocin and amniotomy as concurrent interventions affect outcomes when used for labour augmentation?
- What are the effects of antispasmodic agents when used as treatment for confirmed delay in the first stage of labour?

4.2 Other research questions

The following research questions are listed in no particular order of priority:

- What are the effects of labour augmentation when used for the treatment of delayed labour in women with scarred uterus (i.e. due to previous caesarean section or previous myomectomy)?
    - » What are the effects of amniotomy alone when used for the treatment of delayed labour in women with scarred uterus?
- What are the effects of herbal medications when used for prevention or treatment of delay in labour?
    - » What are the effects of interventions to reduce the use of herbal medications in labour?
- What is the safest maximum dose of oxytocin for labour augmentation?
- What are the effects of the various methods of labour augmentation when used for the treatment of delayed labour in multiparous compared to the nulliparous women?
- What is the safest and most effective incremental rate of oxytocin infusion for labour augmentation?

5. Dissemination and implementation of the guideline

The ultimate goal of this guideline is to improve the quality of care and health outcomes related to labour augmentation. Therefore, the dissemination and implementation of this guideline are crucial steps that should be undertaken by the international community and local health services. The WHO Department of Reproductive Health and Research has adopted a formal knowledge-to-action framework for the dissemination, adaptation and implementation of guidelines (12). In addition to this framework, a list of priority actions was established during the WHO technical consultation for this guideline, and this list will be used by WHO and other partners to foster the dissemination and implementation of this guideline.

5.1 Guideline dissemination and evaluation

The recommendations in this guideline will be disseminated through a broad network of international partners, including WHO country and regional offices, ministries of health, professional organizations, WHO collaborating centres, other United Nations agencies, and nongovernmental organizations. They will also be published on the WHO website[4] and in The *WHO Reproductive Health Library*[5] where they will be accompanied by an independent critical appraisal based on the AGREE instrument (Appraisal of Guidelines Research and Evaluation).[6] A policy brief will also be developed for a wide range of policy-makers, programme managers and clinicians, and then disseminated through WHO country offices.

---

4 Available at: www.who.int/reproductivehealth/topics/maternal_perinatal/augmentation-labour
5 Available at: www.who.int/rhl
6 Available at: http://www.agreecollaboration.org/instrument

5.2 Guideline implementation

The successful introduction of evidence-based policies related to augmentation of labour into national programmes and health services depends on well-planned and participatory consensus-driven processes of adaptation and implementation. These processes may include the development or revision of existing national guidelines or protocols based on this document.

The recommendations contained in the present guideline should be adapted into locally appropriate documents that are able to meet the specific needs of each country and its national health service. Modifications to the recommendations, where necessary, should be limited to weak recommendations, and justifications for any changes should be made in an explicit and transparent manner.

An enabling environment should be created for the use of these recommendations, including changes in the behaviour of health care practitioners and managers to enable the implementation of these evidence-based practices (for example, providing screens for a woman and her birth companion to ensure privacy). Local professional societies may play important roles in this process, and an all-inclusive and participatory process should be encouraged. The WHO Department of Reproductive Health and Research has published specific guidance on the introduction of WHO's reproductive health guidelines and tools into national programmes *(39)*.

6. Applicability issues

6.1 Anticipated impact on the organization of care and resources

The evidence-based practice of augmentation of labour can be achieved with the use of relatively inexpensive medicines and measures. However, the Guideline Development Group noted that the following issues should be considered before the recommendations made in this current guideline are applied:

- Women undergoing augmentation of labour, particularly with oxytocin, should not be left unattended.
- Where oxytocin is used for augmentation, the intravenous infusion rate should be closely monitored. This caution is extremely crucial in settings where gravity drips are used to deliver intravenous infusion.
- In settings where oxytocin is used, attention should be paid to the oxytocin cold chain (i.e. the requirements of a temperature-controlled supply chain).
- Augmentation of labour should be carried out at health-care facilities where there are appropriate resources to regularly monitor fetal heart rate, treat potential adverse effects of the procedure (e.g. tocolysis for hyperstimulation), and manage failure to achieve vaginal birth, including through caesarean section.

6.2 Monitoring and evaluating the guideline implementation

The implementation of the recommendations in this guideline should be monitored at the health service level. Interrupted time series, clinical audits or criterion-based clinical audits could be used to obtain data related to labour augmentation practices. Clearly defined review criteria and indicators are needed and these could be associated with locally agreed targets. In this context, the following indicators are suggested:

1. Augmented labour as a proportion of all births, calculated as the number of women undergoing augmentation of labour divided by the total number of births over a defined period of time.

2. Vaginal birth rate among women undergoing labour augmentation for delay in active labour, calculated as the number of vaginal births in women undergoing augmentation of labour divided by the total number of women undergoing augmentation of labour.

3. Caesarean section rate among women undergoing labour augmentation for delay in active labour, calculated as the number of caesarean sections in women undergoing augmentation of labour divided by the total number of women undergoing augmentation of labour.

The first indicator provides an overall assessment of the use of augmentation of labour while the second and third indicators provide an evaluation of the success of the procedure and could be compared to the overall caesarean section rate in the local context. The use of other locally developed indicators (e.g. use of practices that are not recommended) may be necessary to obtain a more complete assessment of the quality of care related to the practice of augmentation of labour.

7. Updating the guideline

In accordance with the concept of WHO's GREAT project *(12)*, which employs a systematic and continuous process of identifying and bridging evidence gaps following guideline implementation, this guideline will be updated five years after publication or following the identification of new evidence that indicates a need to revise these recommendations. WHO welcomes suggestions regarding additional questions for inclusion in the updated guideline. Please email your suggestions to: reproductivehealth@who.int.

References

1. Ronel D, Wiznitzer A, Sergienko R, Zlotnik A, Sheiner E. Trends, risk factors and pregnancy outcome in women with uterine rupture. *Arch Gynecol Obstet.* 2012;285(2):317–21.

2. McClure EM, Saleem S, Pasha O, Goldenberg RL. Stillbirth in developing countries: a review of causes, risk factors and prevention strategies. *J Matern Fetal Neonatal Med.* 2009;22(3):183–90.

3. Kjaergaard H, Olsen J, Ottesen B, Dykes AK. Incidence and outcomes of dystocia in the active phase of labor in term nulliparous women with spontaneous labor onset. *Acta Obstet Gynecol Scand.* 2009;88(4):402–7.

4. Boyle A, Reddy UM, Landy HJ, Huang CC, Driggers RW, Laughon SK. Primary cesarean delivery in the United States. *Obstet Gynecol.* 2013;122(1):33–40.

5. O Driscoll K, Foley M, MacDonald D. Active management of labour as an alternative to caesarean section for dystocia. *Obstet Gynecol.* 1984;63(4):485–90.

6. Brown HC, Paranjothy S, Dowswell T, Thomas J. Package of care for active management in labour for reducing caesarean section rates in low-risk women. *Cochrane Database Syst Rev.* 2013;(9):CD004907.

7. Bernitz S, Oian P, Rolland R, Sandvik L, Blix E. Oxytocin and dystocia as risk factors for adverse birth outcomes: a cohort of low-risk nulliparous women. *Midwifery.* 2014;30(3):364–70.

8. Selin L, Almström E, Wallin G, Berg M. Use and abuse of oxytocin for augmentation of labor. *Acta Obstet Gynecol Scand.* 2009;88(12):1352–7.

9. Jonsson M, Nordén-Lindeberg S, Ostlund I, Hanson U. Acidemia at birth, related to obstetric characteristics and to oxytocin use, during the last two hours of labor. *Acta Obstet Gynecol Scand.* 2008;87(7):745–50.

10. Zhang J, Branch DW, Ramirez MM, Laughon SK, Reddy U, Hoffman M, et al. Oxytocin regimen for labor augmentation, labor progression, perinatal outcomes. *Obstet Gynecol.* 2011;118(2 Pt 1):249–56.

11. *WHO recommendations for induction of labour.* Geneva: World Health Organization; 2011 (http://whqlibdoc.who.int/publications/2011/9789241501156_eng.pdf, accessed 26 March 2014).

12. *Science-driven innovations for combating maternal and perinatal ill-health: the G.R.E.A.T project.* Geneva: World Health Organization; 2010 (http://www.who.int/reproductivehealth/topics/best_practices/Great_Project_2010.pdf, accessed 26 March 2014).

13. WHO handbook for guideline development. Geneva: World Health Organization; 2012 (http://apps.who.int/iris/bitstream/10665/75146/1/9789241548441_eng.pdf, accessed 26 March 2014).

14. Andrews J, Guyatt G, Oxman AD, Alderson P, Dahm P, Falck-Ytter Y, et al. GRADE guidelines: 14. Going from evidence to recommendations: the significance and presentation of recommendations. *J Clin Epidemiol.* 2013;66(7):719–25.

15. Lavender T, Hart A, Smyth RMD. Effect of partogram use on outcomes for women in spontaneous labour at term. *Cochrane Database Syst Rev.* 2013;(7):CD005461.

16. Downe S, Gill GML, Dahlen, Dahlen HG, Singata M. Routine vaginal examinations for assessing progress of labour to improve outcomes for women and babies at term. *Cochrane Database Syst Rev.* 2013;(7):CD010088.

17. Wei S, Wo BL, Qi HP, Xu H, Luo ZC, Roy C, Fraser WD. Early amniotomy and early oxytocin for prevention of, or therapy for, delay in first stage spontaneous labour compared with routine care. *Cochrane Database Syst Rev.* 2013;(8):CD006794.

18. Costley PL, East CE. Oxytocin augmentation of labour in women with epidural analgesia for reducing operative deliveries. *Cochrane Database Syst Rev.* 2013;(7):CD009241.

19. Smyth RMD, Markham C, Dowswell T. Amniotomy for shortening spontaneous labour. *Cochrane Database Syst Rev.* 2013;(6):CD006167.

20. Rohwer AC, Khondowe O, Young T. Antispasmodics for labour. *Cochrane Database Syst Rev.* 2013;(6):CD009243.

21. Anim-Somuah M, Smyth RMD, Jones L. Epidural versus non-epidural or no analgesia in labour. *Cochrane Database Syst Rev.* 2011;(12):CD000331.

22. Novikova N, Cluver C. Local anaesthetic nerve block for pain management in labour. *Cochrane Database Syst Rev.* 2012;(4):CD009200.

23. Simmons SW, Taghizadeh N, Dennis AT, Hughes D, Cyna AM. Combined spinal-epidural versus epidural analgesia in labour. *Cochrane Database Syst Rev.* 2012;(10):CD003401.

24. Dowswell T, Bedwell C, Lavender T, Neilson JP. Transcutaneous electrical nerve stimulation (TENS) for pain management in labour. *Cochrane Database Syst Rev.* 2009;(2):CD007214.

25. Smith CA, Levett KM, Collins CT, Crowther CA. Relaxation techniques for pain management in labour. *Cochrane Database Syst Rev.* 2011;(12):CD009514.

26. Smith CA, Collins CT, Crowther CA, Levett KM. Acupuncture or acupressure for pain management in labour. *Cochrane Database Syst Rev.* 2011;(7):CD009232.

27. Madden K, Middleton P, Cyna AM, Matthewson M, Jones L. Hypnosis for pain management during labour and childbirth. *Cochrane Database Syst Rev.* 2012;(11):CD009356.

28. Smith CA, Collins CT, Crowther CA. Aromatherapy for pain management in labour. *Cochrane Database Syst Rev.* 2011;(7):CD009215.

29. Barragán Loayza IM, Solà I, Juandó Prats C. Biofeedback for pain management during labour. *Cochrane Database Syst Rev.* 2011;(6):CD006168.

30. Dawood F, Dowswell T, Quenby S. Intravenous fluids for reducing the duration of labour in low risk nulliparous women. *Cochrane Database Syst Rev.* 2013;(6):CD007715.

31. Singata M, Tranmer J, Gyte GML. Restricting oral fluid and food intake during labour. *Cochrane Database Syst Rev.* 2013;(8):CD003930.

32. Lawrence A, Lewis L, Hofmeyr GJ, Styles C. Maternal positions and mobility during first stage labour. *Cochrane Database Syst Rev.* 2013;(8):CD003934.

33. Hodnett ED, Gates S, Hofmeyr GJ, Sakala C. Continuous support for women during childbirth. *Cochrane Database Syst Rev.* 2013;(7):CD003766.

34. Reveiz L, Gaitán HG, Cuervo LG. Enemas during labour. *Cochrane Database Syst Rev.* 2013;(5):CD000330.

35. Bugg GJ, Siddiqui F, Thornton JG. Oxytocin versus no treatment or delayed treatment for slow progress in the first stage of spontaneous labour. *Cochrane Database Syst Rev.* 2013;(6):CD007123.

36. Kenyon S, Tokumasu H, Dowswell T, Pledge D, Mori R. High-dose versus low-dose oxytocin for augmentation of delayed labour. *Cochrane Database Syst Rev.* 2013;(7):CD007201.

37. Vogel JP, West HM, Dowswell T. Titrated oral misoprostol for augmenting labour to improve maternal and neonatal outcomes. *Cochrane Database Syst Rev.* 2013;(9):CD010648.

38. Bakker JJH, Janssen PF, van Halem K, van der Goes BY, Papatsonis DNM, van der Post JAM, et al. Internal versus external tocodynamometry during induced or augmented labour. *Cochrane Database Syst Rev.* 2013;(8):CD006947.

39. *Introducing WHO's sexual and reproductive health guidelines and tools into national programmes: principles and processes of adaptation and implementation.* Geneva: World Health Organization; 2007 (WHO/RHR/07.9; http://www.who.int/reproductivehealth/publications/general/RHR_07_09/en/index.html, accessed 26 March 2014).

Annex 1. External experts and WHO staff involved in the preparation of the guideline

A. Participants at the WHO technical consultation on augmentation of labour

1. Guideline Development Group (WHO external partners)

Professor Hany Abdel-Aleem
Department of Obstetrics and Gynecology
Faculty of Medicine
Assiut University
71515 Assiut
Egypt

Professor Michel Boulvain
Maternité-HUG
Service d'obstétrique
Bd. de la Cluse
Geneve 1211
Switzerland

Dr Yap-Seng Chong
Associate Professor
Department of Obstetrics and Gynaecology
Yong Loo Lin School of Medicine
National University of Singapore
Singapore

Professor Arri Coomarasamy
University of Birmingham
Birmingham Women's Hospital Foundation Trust
Academic Unit, 3rd Floor, Mindelsohn Way
Edgbaston, Birmingham B15 2TG
United Kingdom

Dr Therese Dowswell
Research Associate
Cochrane Pregnancy and Childbirth Group
Department of Women's and Children's Health
The University of Liverpool
Liverpool Women's NHS Foundation Trust
Crown Street, Liverpool, L8 7SS
United Kingdom

Dr Bukola Fawole
Senior Lecturer
College of Medicine
University of Ibadan
Ibadan
Nigeria

Dr Atf Ghérissi
Assistant Professor
Education Science
High School for Sciences and Health Techniques of Tunis
Tunis-El Manar University
Tunis
Tunisia

Professor Justus Hofmeyr
Department of Obstetrics and Gynaecology
Frere Maternity Hospital
P Bag X9047
East London
South Africa

Ms Rachael Lockey
Technical Midwife Adviser
International Confederation of Midwives
Laam van Meerdervoort 70, 2517 AN
The Hague
The Netherlands

Professor Jiji Elizabeth Mathews
Christian Medical College and Hospital
Department of Obstetrics and Gynaecology
Unit 5, Ida Scudder Road
Vellore 632004
India

Dr Kidza Yvonne Mugerwa
Honorary Lecturer
Department of Obstetrics and Gynaecology
School of Medicine, College of Health Sciences
Makerere University
Kampala
Uganda

Professor Zahida Qureshi
Department of Obstetrics and Gynaecology
University of Nairobi
Kenya

Professor Hora Soltani
Professor of Maternal and Infant Health
Centre for Health and Social Care Research
Sheffield Hallam University
32 Collegiate Crescent, S10 2BP
United Kingdom

Dr Helen West
Research Assistant
Cochrane Pregnancy and Childbirth Group
Department of Women's and Children's Health
The University of Liverpool
Liverpool Women's NHS Foundation Trust
Crown Street, Liverpool L8 7SS
United Kingdom

2. Observer

Ms Deborah Armbruster
Senior Maternal and Newborn Health Advisor
Bureau for Global Health
Office of Health, Infectious Diseases and Nutrition (HIDN)
Maternal and Child Health Division (MCH)
United States Agency for International Development
Washington DC
USA

3. WHO country and regional offices

Dr Gunta Lazdane
Programme Manager
Sexual and Reproductive Health
WHO Regional Office for Europe
Copenhagen
Denmark

Dr Léopold Ouedraogo
Regional Adviser
Research and Programme Development in Reproductive Health
Health Promotion Cluster
WHO Regional Office for Africa
BP. 06 Brazzaville
Republic of Congo

Dr Suzanne Serruya
Regional Adviser on Reproductive Health
Latin American Centre for Perinatology, Women and Reproductive Health
WHO Regional Office for the Americas/Pan American Health Organization (PAHO)
Montevideo
Uruguay

Dr Martin Weber
Regional Adviser
Making Pregnancy Safer and Reproductive Health
WHO Regional Office for South-East Asia
World Health House, Indraprastha Estate
Mahatma Gandhi Road
New Delhi 11000
India

4. WHO Secretariat

Dr Marleen Temmerman
Director
Department of Reproductive Health and Research

Dr Metin Gülmezoglu
Coordinator
Maternal and Perinatal Health & Preventing Unsafe Abortion
Department of Reproductive Health and Research

Dr Matthews Mathai
Coordinator
Epidemiology, Monitoring and Evaluation
Department of Maternal, Newborn, Child and Adolescent Health

Dr Olufemi Oladapo
Medical Officer
Maternal and Perinatal Health & Preventing Unsafe Abortion
Department of Reproductive Health and Research

Ms Mariana Widmer
Technical Officer
Maternal and Perinatal Health & Preventing Unsafe Abortion
Department of Reproductive Health and Research

Ms Frances McConville
Technical Officer
Policy, Planning and Programmes
Department of Maternal, Newborn, Child and Adolescent Health

Dr Joshua Vogel
Technical Officer
Maternal and Perinatal Health & Preventing Unsafe Abortion
Department of Reproductive Health and Research

B. Guideline Steering Group

Dr A. Metin Gülmezoglu
(WHO Department of Reproductive Health and Research)

Dr Matthews Mathai
(WHO Department of Maternal, Newborn, Child and Adolescent Health)

Dr Olufemi Oladapo
(WHO Department of Reproductive Health and Research)

Dr João Paulo Souza
(WHO Department of Reproductive Health and Research)

Ms Mariana Widmer
(WHO Department of Reproductive Health and Research)

C. External Review Group

Dr Edgardo Abalos
Vice Director
Centro Rosarino de Estudios Perinatales
Rosario
Argentina

Professor Pisake Lumbiganon
Department of Obstetrics and Gynaecology
Faculty of Medicine
Khon Kaen University
Khon Kaen
Thailand

Professor Suneeta Mittal
Officer-in-Charge
WHO Collaborating Centre for Research on Human Reproduction
All India Institute of Medical Sciences
New Delhi
India

Annex 2. Critical and important outcomes for decision-making

Critical maternal outcomes

- Uterine hyperstimulation with fetal heart rate changes necessitating intervention
- Maternal mortality
- Total duration of labour
- Serious maternal morbidity
- Postpartum haemorrhage
- Vaginal birth not achieved within 24 hours, from onset of labour
- Duration of the first stage of labour
- Caesarean section for fetal distress

Critical infant outcomes

- Stillbirth or neonatal death
- Neonatal morbidity, excluding fatal malformations (e.g. seizures, birth asphyxia)
- Apgar score < 7 at five minutes
- Cord blood arterial pH < 7.1
- Birth trauma (e.g. cephalhaematoma, Erb's palsy, bone fracture)

Important maternal outcomes

- Hyperstimulation of labour
- Dysfunctional labour
- Spontaneous vaginal birth
- Blood transfusion
- Caesarean section for prolonged labour
- Duration of second stage of labour
- Chorioamnionitis
- Adverse effects of amniotomy: umbilical cord prolapse, infection
- Time interval between amniotomy and birth of baby
- Epidural analgesia
- Third and fourth degree tears
- Duration of rupture of the membranes at the time of delivery
- Rate of cervical dilatation (cm/hr)
- Instrumental vaginal birth
- Postnatal depression
- Pulmonary embolism
- Satisfaction with childbirth experience
- Antepartum haemorrhage
- Prolonged hospital stay
- Postpartum re-hospitalization
- Maternal health service utilization (cost)
- Pyrexia

Important infant outcomes

- Admission to neonatal intensive care unit
- Need for intubation at delivery
- Childhood disability
- Prolonged stay for infants
- Readmission to hospital for infants
- Jaundice

Annex 3. Summary of the considerations related to the strength of the recommendations (balance worksheets)

These and all EB tables are presented in the Evidence base document, available at: www.who.int/reproductivehealth/topics/maternal_perinatal/augmentation-labour

Box 1. Summary of considerations related to the strength of the recommendations (Recommendations Nos. 1–5)

Recommendation No.	1	2	3	4	5
Intervention	Partograph for monitoring the progress in labour	Routine vaginal examination for assessing progress of labour	Package of care for active management of labour	Early amniotomy and early oxytocin for preventing delay	Oxytocin augmentation for women under epidural analgesia
Quality of the evidence	☐ High ☐ Moderate ☐ Low ☒ Very low	☐ High ☐ Moderate ☐ Low ☒ Very low	☐ High ☐ Moderate ☒ Low ☐ Very low	☐ High ☐ Moderate ☐ Low ☒ Very low	☐ High ☐ Moderate ☒ Low ☐ Very low
Values and preferences	☒ No significant variability ☐ Significant variability	☐ No significant variability ☒ Significant variability	☐ No significant variability ☒ Significant variability	☐ No significant variability ☒ Significant variability	☐ No significant variability ☒ Significant variability
Absolute magnitude of effect	☐ Large effect (RR>2 or RR<0.5) ☒ Small effect (0.5<RR<2)	☐ Large effect (RR>2 or RR<0.5) ☒ Small effect (0.5<RR<2)	☐ Large effect (RR>2 or RR<0.5) ☒ Small effect (0.5<RR<2)	☐ Large effect (RR>2 or RR<0.5) ☒ Small effect (0.5<RR<2)	☐ Large effect (RR>2 or RR<0.5) ☒ Small effect (0.5<RR<2)
Balance of benefits versus disadvantages	☒ Benefits outweigh disadvantages ☐ Benefits and disadvantages are balanced ☐ Disadvantages outweigh benefits	☒ Benefits outweigh disadvantages ☐ Benefits and disadvantages are balanced ☐ Disadvantages outweigh benefits	☐ Benefits outweigh disadvantages ☒ Benefits and disadvantages are balanced ☐ Disadvantages outweigh benefits	☐ Benefits outweigh disadvantages ☒ Benefits and disadvantages are balanced ☐ Disadvantages outweigh benefits	☐ Benefits outweigh disadvantages ☒ Benefits and disadvantages are balanced ☐ Disadvantages outweigh benefits
Resource use	☒ Less resource intensive ☐ More resource intensive	☒ Less resource intensive ☐ More resource intensive	☐ Less resource intensive ☒ More resource intensive	☐ Less resource intensive ☒ More resource intensive	☐ Less resource intensive ☒ More resource intensive
Feasibility	☒ Yes, globally ☐ Yes, conditionally	☐ Yes, globally ☒ Yes, conditionally	☐ Yes, globally ☒ Yes, conditionally	☐ Yes, globally ☒ Yes, conditionally	☐ Yes, globally ☒ Yes, conditionally
Recommendation direction	☒ In favour of the intervention ☐ Against the intervention	☒ In favour of the intervention ☐ Against the intervention	☐ In favour of the intervention ☒ Against the intervention	☐ In favour of the intervention ☒ Against the intervention	☐ In favour of the intervention ☒ Against the intervention
Overall ranking	☒ Strong recommendation ☐ Weak recommendation	☐ Strong recommendation ☒ Weak recommendation	☐ Strong recommendation ☒ Weak recommendation	☐ Strong recommendation ☒ Weak recommendation	☐ Strong recommendation ☒ Weak recommendation

Box 2. Summary of considerations related to the strength of the recommendations (Recommendations Nos. 6–10)

Recommendation No.	6	7	8	9	10
Intervention	Amniotomy alone for preventing delay in labour	Antispasmodics for preventing delay in labour	Effect of pain relief on duration of labour and oxytocin augmentation	Intravenous fluids for shortening the duration of labour	Oral fluid and food intake during labour
Quality of the evidence	☐ High ☐ Moderate ☐ Low ☒ Very low	☐ High ☐ Moderate ☐ Low ☒ Very low	☐ High ☐ Moderate ☐ Low ☒ Very low	☐ High ☐ Moderate ☐ Low ☒ Very low	☐ High ☐ Moderate ☐ Low ☒ Very low
Values and preferences	☐ No significant variability ☒ Significant variability	☐ No significant variability ☒ Significant variability	☐ No significant variability ☒ Significant variability	☐ No significant variability ☒ Significant variability	☒ No significant variability ☐ Significant variability
Absolute magnitude of effect	☐ Large effect (RR>2 or RR<0.5) ☒ Small effect (0.5<RR<2)	☐ Large effect (RR>2 or RR<0.5) ☒ Small effect (0.5<RR<2)	☐ Large effect (RR>2 or RR<0.5) ☒ Small effect (0.5<RR<2)	☐ Large effect (RR>2 or RR<0.5) ☒ Small effect (0.5<RR<2)	☐ Large effect (RR>2 or RR<0.5) ☒ Small effect (0.5<RR<2)
Balance of benefits versus disadvantages	☐ Benefits outweigh disadvantages ☒ Benefits and disadvantages are balanced ☐ Disadvantages outweigh benefits	☐ Benefits outweigh disadvantages ☒ Benefits and disadvantages are balanced ☐ Disadvantages outweigh benefits	☐ Benefits outweigh disadvantages ☒ Benefits and disadvantages are balanced ☐ Disadvantages outweigh benefits	☐ Benefits outweigh disadvantages ☐ Benefits and disadvantages are balanced ☒ Disadvantages outweigh benefits	☐ Benefits outweigh disadvantages ☒ Benefits and disadvantages are balanced ☐ Disadvantages outweigh benefits
Resource use	☒ Less resource intensive ☐ More resource intensive	☒ Less resource intensive ☐ More resource intensive	☐ Less resource intensive ☒ More resource intensive	☐ Less resource intensive ☒ More resource intensive	☒ Less resource intensive ☐ More resource intensive
Feasibility	☐ Yes, globally ☒ Yes, conditionally	☒ Yes, globally ☐ Yes, conditionally	☐ Yes, globally ☒ Yes, conditionally	☐ Yes, globally ☒ Yes, conditionally	Yes, globally ☒ Yes, conditionally
Recommendation direction	☐ In favour of the intervention ☒ Against the intervention	☐ In favour of the intervention ☒ Against the intervention	☐ In favour of the intervention ☒ Against the intervention	☐ In favour of the intervention ☒ Against the intervention	☒ In favour of the intervention ☐ Against the intervention
Overall ranking	☐ Strong recommendation ☒ Weak recommendation	☐ Strong recommendation ☒ Weak recommendation	☐ Strong recommendation ☒ Weak recommendation	☒ Strong recommendation ☐ Weak recommendation	☐ Strong recommendation ☒ Weak recommendation

Box 3. Summary of considerations related to the strength of the recommendations (Recommendations Nos. 11–15)

Recommendation	11	12	13	14	15
Intervention	Maternal position and mobility during labour	Continuous companionship during labour	Routine enema for improving labour outcomes	Oxytocin alone for treating delay in labour	Early amniotomy and early oxytocin for treating delay
Quality of the evidence	☐ High ☐ Moderate ☐ Low ☒ Very low	☐ High ☒ Moderate ☐ Low ☐ Very low	☐ High ☐ Moderate ☐ Low ☒ Very low	☐ High ☐ Moderate ☐ Low ☒ Very low	☐ High ☐ Moderate ☐ Low ☒ Very low
Values and preferences	☐ No significant variability ☒ Significant variability	☐ No significant variability ☒ Significant variability	☐ No significant variability ☒ Significant variability	☒ No significant variability ☐ Significant variability	☐ No significant variability ☒ Significant variability
Absolute magnitude of effect	☐ Large effect (RR>2 or RR<0.5) ☒ Small effect (0.5<RR<2)	☐ Large effect (RR>2 or RR<0.5) ☒ Small effect (0.5<RR<2)	☐ Large effect (RR>2 or RR<0.5) ☒ Small effect (0.5<RR<2)	☐ Large effect (RR>2 or RR<0.5) ☒ Small effect (0.5<RR<2)	☐ Large effect (RR>2 or RR<0.5) ☒ Small effect (0.5<RR<2)
Balance of benefits versus disadvantages	☒ Benefits outweigh disadvantages ☐ Benefits and disadvantages are balanced ☐ Disadvantages outweigh benefits	☒ Benefits outweigh disadvantages ☐ Benefits and disadvantages are balanced ☐ Disadvantages outweigh benefits	☐ Benefits outweigh disadvantages ☐ Benefits and disadvantages are balanced ☒ Disadvantages outweigh benefits	☐ Benefits outweigh disadvantages ☒ Benefits and disadvantages are balanced ☐ Disadvantages outweigh benefits	☐ Benefits outweigh disadvantages ☐ Benefits and disadvantages are balanced ☒ Disadvantages outweigh benefits
Resource use	☒ Less resource intensive ☐ More resource intensive	☒ Less resource intensive ☐ More resource intensive	☐ Less resource intensive ☒ More resource intensive	☒ Less resource intensive ☐ More resource intensive	☐ Less resource intensive ☒ More resource intensive
Feasibility	☒ Yes, globally ☐ Yes, conditionally	☐ Yes, globally ☒ Yes, conditionally	☐ Yes, globally ☒ Yes, conditionally	☒ Yes, globally ☐ Yes, conditionally	☐ Yes, globally ☒ Yes, conditionally
Recommendation direction	☒ In favour of the intervention ☐ Against the intervention	☒ In favour of the intervention ☐ Against the intervention	☐ In favour of the intervention ☒ Against the intervention	☒ In favour of the intervention ☐ Against the intervention	☐ In favour of the intervention ☒ Against the intervention
Overall ranking	☒ Strong recommendation ☐ Weak recommendation	☒ Strong recommendation ☐ Weak recommendation	☒ Strong recommendation ☐ Weak recommendation	☐ Strong recommendation ☒ Weak recommendation	☒ Strong recommendation ☐ Weak recommendation

Box 4. Summary of considerations related to the strength of the recommendations (Recommendations Nos. 16–20)

Recommendation	16	17	18	19	20
Intervention	High starting and increment oxytocin dosage regimen for augmentation	Oral misoprostol for labour augmentation	Amniotomy alone for treatment of delay	Amniotomy and oxytocin for treatment of delay	Internal versus external tocodynamometry in augmented labour
Quality of the evidence	☐ High ☐ Moderate ☐ Low ☒ Very low	☐ High ☐ Moderate ☐ Low ☒ Very low	☐ High ☐ Moderate ☐ Low ☒ Very low	☐ High ☐ Moderate ☐ Low ☒ Very low	☐ High ☐ Moderate ☐ Low ☒ Very low
Values and preferences	☐ No significant variability ☒ Significant variability	☒ No significant variability ☐ Significant variability	☐ No significant variability ☒ Significant variability	☐ No significant variability ☒ Significant variability	☐ No significant variability ☒ Significant variability
Absolute magnitude of effect	☐ Large effect (RR>2 or RR<0.5) ☒ Small effect (0.5<RR<2)	☐ Large effect (RR>2 or RR<0.5) ☒ Small effect (0.5<RR<2)	☐ Large effect (RR>2 or RR<0.5) ☒ Small effect (0.5<RR<2)	☐ Large effect (RR>2 or RR<0.5) ☒ Small effect (0.5<RR<2)	☐ Large effect (RR>2 or RR<0.5) ☒ Small effect (0.5<RR<2)
Balance of benefits versus disadvantages	☐ Benefits outweigh disadvantages ☐ Benefits and disadvantages are balanced ☒ Disadvantages outweigh benefits	☐ Benefits outweigh disadvantages ☐ Benefits and disadvantages are balanced ☒ Disadvantages outweigh benefits	☐ Benefits outweigh disadvantages ☒ Benefits and disadvantages are balanced ☐ Disadvantages outweigh benefits	☐ Benefits outweigh disadvantages ☒ Benefits and disadvantages are balanced ☐ Disadvantages outweigh benefits	☐ Benefits outweigh disadvantages ☒ Benefits and disadvantages are balanced ☐ Disadvantages outweigh benefits
Resource use	☐ Less resource intensive ☒ More resource intensive	☒ Less resource intensive ☐ More resource intensive	☒ Less resource intensive ☐ More resource intensive	☒ Less resource intensive ☐ More resource intensive	☐ Less resource intensive ☒ More resource intensive
Feasibility	☐ Yes, globally ☒ Yes, conditionally	☐ Yes, globally ☒ Yes, conditionally	☒ Yes, globally ☐ Yes, conditionally	☒ Yes, globally ☐ Yes, conditionally	☐ Yes, globally ☒ Yes, conditionally
Recommendation direction	☐ In favour of the intervention ☒ Against the intervention	☐ In favour of the intervention ☒ Against the intervention	☐ In favour of the intervention ☒ Against the intervention	☒ In favour of the intervention ☐ Against the intervention	☐ In favour of the intervention ☒ Against the intervention
Overall ranking	☐ Strong recommendation ☒ Weak recommendation	☐ Strong recommendation ☒ Weak recommendation	☐ Strong recommendation ☒ Weak recommendation	☐ Strong recommendation ☒ Weak recommendation	☐ Strong recommendation ☒ Weak recommendation

Box 5. Template for the summary of considerations related to the strength of the recommendations with explanations for completing the template

Recommendation	Which recommendation?	
Intervention	What is the intervention?	
Quality of the evidence	☐ High	The higher the quality of the evidence, the stronger the recommendation.
	☐ Moderate	If the quality of the evidence is low or very low, consider more carefully the other criteria below in deciding the strength of the recommendation.
	☐ Low	
	☐ Very low	
Values and preferences	☐ No significant variability	This refers to values placed by health workers, policy-makers, patients and other stakeholders on the intended outcomes of the intervention.
	☐ Significant variability	If there is wide variability between the values and preferences of various stakeholders, the intervention is less likely to have a strong recommendation.
Magnitude of effect in critical outcomes	☐ Large effect (RR>2 or RR<0.5)	This refers to the potential of the intervention to have large effects. The effects can be enhanced by being combined with other interventions. Consider which potential associations (or "bundles") can enhance effects.
	☐ Small effect (0.5<RR<2)	The larger the potential effects and the longer the time period of the potential effects, the more likely the intervention is to have a strong recommendation.
Balance of benefits versus disadvantages	☐ Benefits outweigh disadvantages	Benefits refer to the intended positive effects of an intervention.
	☐ Benefits and disadvantages are balanced	Disadvantages refer to the potentially negative effects of an intervention as well as its unintended effects.
	☐ Disadvantages outweigh benefits	The fewer potential negative effects there are, the more likely the intervention is to receive a strong recommendation.
Resource use	☐ Less resource intensive	The resources needed for the implementation of a recommendation may include financial resources, human resources, and infrastructure or equipment. Ideally, the cost of the benefits of an intervention should be reasonable, affordable and sustainable. It should be remembered that capital costs, such as those required for infrastructural development, may be high initially but may also yield long-term benefits.
	☐ More resource intensive	Generally, interventions that incur higher incremental or recurrent costs are less likely to be strongly recommended.
Feasibility	☐ Yes, globally	Political commitment and wide stakeholder engagement are prerequisites for interventions. The 'technical' feasibility of interventions also depends on sufficiently functional organizational and institutional structures to manage, follow through, and monitor the implementation of the recommendation. The elements of technical feasibility vary considerably by country and by context; where these elements are likely to be functional across a wide variety of settings it is more likely that the intervention will receive a strong recommendation.
	☐ Yes, conditionally	
Recommendation direction	☐ In favour of the intervention	
	☐ Against the intervention	
Overall ranking	☐ Strong recommendation	Strength of the recommendation.
	☐ Weak recommendation	